Silica Water the Secret of Healthy Longevity in the Aluminum Age

Author: Dr. Dennis N. Crouse, BSc Biochemistry, - Harvard College, Ph.D. Organic Chemistry - Harvard University Chemistry Department, Post-graduate courses: Understanding Dementia - Wicking Faculty of Health, University of Tasmania, Fundamentals of Neuroscience - Harvard.

Printed in the United States of America

Fourth Edition, 2022

ISBN 978-1727336740

Etiological Publishing

Dedication

This book is dedicated to my mother and father: Beulah J. and Norman G. Crouse

Both of whom encouraged me to observe nature and discover why on my own

Forward

"If there is magic on this planet, it is contained in the water."

Loren C. Eiseley – The Immense Journey 1946

We have all heard that we can learn from our elders. By taking this advice and looking at geographic regions on earth where the density of centenarians is higher than normal, we have learned from the elders living there the secret of healthy longevity. Amazingly there is magic in their drinking water and in some of the food they eat! The science behind this magic and how we can use it to achieve our own individual and cultural healthy longevity is the subject of this book. We need this magic more now than ever before as we are living in the Aluminum Age in which the neurotoxin aluminum is being increasingly put in our food, drinking water, kitchen ware, pharmaceuticals, vaccines, colored candy, cosmetics, and even the air we inhale. If you are interested in finding out what is behind the curtain of this magic, join me in the exciting search for the secret of healthy longevity in the aluminum age.

Acknowledgements

I appreciate the support and encouragement of my wife Laurie Adamson who has been an immense help in the search for information. I thank Dr. Chris Exley and those who have worked with Chris for showing me how to help my mother heal her Alzheimer's. Special thanks to all the people who have posted the anecdotal information at group sites and pages on Facebook that appears in this book. I have kept the names of sources of this very personal information anonymous. You and your children are the true pioneers who are shinning the light for hopefully many more to follow you out of the darkness of the Aluminum Age. Special thanks to Dr. Carol T. Walsh for her editing and useful comments. Thanks to Dr. Christopher Shaw for his useful comments. Thanks to Jere Beasley for his edits. Thanks to both Paul Watling for fact finding and Bill Hamilton for the shortened Silicade recipe. Thanks to Melissa Easter for her useful comments.

Table of Contents

The information presented in this book with gray backgrounds goes into greater depth on relevant topics. Reading this information is not required to understand the thesis and conclusions of this book.

About the Title

This book is the fourth edition of my popular 2018 book by a similar title. In addition to a new title and cover, there is updated anecdotal information on silica water's efficacy for treating Alzheimer's disease in Chapter 5, new analytical data on high silica waters in Appendix I and IV, and more data on TRS and Epson salt baths in Chapter 7.

The "aluminum age" was first mentioned in an 1893 editorial by the British weekly the Spectator that was inspired by Alfred Gilbert's aluminum statue of Eros[452]. This was the first London statue to be cast in aluminum. The statue was unveiled in 1893 and is currently located on the southeastern side of Piccadilly Circus. Gilbert said the statue represented *"the blindfolded Love sending forth indiscriminately, yet with purpose, his missile of kindness, always with the swiftness of the bird has from its wings"*. The editor for the Spectator was more enamored with aluminum and hailed aluminum as *"beautiful to the eye, whiter than silver, and indestructible by contact with air, ... strong, elastic, and so light that the imagination almost refuses to conceive it as a metal."* The editor concluded just as *"the world has seen its age of stone, its age of bronze, and its age of iron, so it may before long have embarked on a new and even more prosperous era – **the age of aluminium**."*[452]

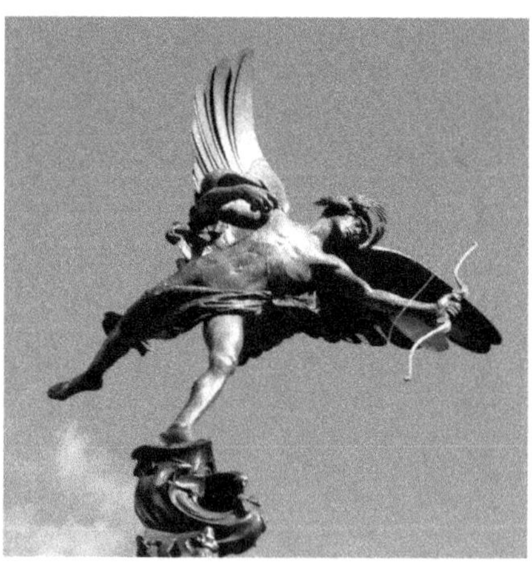

Love for aluminum at first sight can be deceiving.

About the Author

My interest in **silica water** was inspired by a desire to help my mother slow the progression of her Alzheimer's disease. My mother was 86 when she lost her short-term memory and was diagnosed with mild cognitive impairment (MCI). The facts that she had MCI and could no longer perform daily tasks such as meal preparation, sewing, and balancing the checkbook, were indications she had Alzheimer's disease. In order to save my mother from the terrible death of end-stage Alzheimer's disease (AD), I devoted myself to studying scientific literature looking for causal factors of AD. My belief was that only by finding a causal factor could I help my mother stop the progression of AD.

After 3 years of reading, I concluded that aluminum is a causal factor of AD and that my mother was being exposed to the following daily sources of aluminum:

- Drinking Water (50mcg/L aluminum and no silica)

- Drip Style Coffee Maker - with aluminum heating element (260mcg/L of aluminum)

- Baking Powder (50mg aluminum per teaspoon)

- Homemade Tomato Juice - made in an aluminum kettle (>1,000mcg/L of aluminum)

I also read Dr. Christopher Exley's work on daily silica water treatments improving cognition in some Alzheimer's patients by facilitating aluminum excretion and hoped this might work for my mother. Luckily my mother and father still had the ability to adapt to change. In other words, they had resiliency and were willing to make lifestyle changes to avoid sources of aluminum. Most importantly they were willing to switch over to drinking silica water (e.g., Fiji water) instead of tap water.

In 2014, my 87-year-old mother, who at the time was diagnosed with MCI, began daily drinking an OSA rich water (i.e., Fiji Water) in an effort to improve her loss of short-term memory. My mother is an *ApoE E4* carrier. After two years of daily drinking the OSA rich water there was both a clearly noticeable and clinically evaluated improvement in my mother's short-term memory at age 89. I was very thankful! Her improved memory allowed my mother to continue to live in her home with only my father's help. Mother drank Fiji water every day in her coffee and tea for 5 years from age 87 to 92. After my father died in early 2019 at age 95, my mother no longer regularly drank Fiji water but continued to live alone in her house to age 94½. Sadly since 2019 her memory resumed its decline.

My research on Alzheimer's disease and ways to prevent it are summarized in my book "Prevent Alzheimer's, Autism, and Stroke with 7 Supplements, 7 Lifestyle Choices, and a Dissolved Mineral"[1]. The dissolved mineral is a water-soluble silica derivative called orthosilicic acid (OSA). The reversal of Alzheimer's symptoms in my mother motivated me to write this book on the health and longevity benefits of silica water.

I was fortunate as a freshman at Harvard to have Dr. Lewis L. Engle Professor of Biological Chemistry at Harvard Medical School as my tutor. During our first meeting Dr. Engle suggested I read a book written almost 40 years earlier by Lawrence J. Henderson Assistant Professor of Biological Chemistry at Harvard University entitled "The Fitness of The Environment". This book describes how the earth's chemical environment made life on earth sustainable. The information in Henderson's book shaped my career path.

Even before graduating from Harvard with a Ph.D. I cofounded a company to detect and quantify toxic chemicals in food. The company's commercial chemical analysis laboratory performed analytical procedures for a wide variety of toxic environmental chemicals. Most of these toxic chemicals are man-made and eroding the fitness of our environment for sustaining life on earth.

Because of my recent research into my mother's Alzheimer's disease, I have now added aluminum to the list of toxic chemicals that are increasing in our diet and accumulating in our brains due to man's influence. Aluminum is a neurotoxin and chronic accumulation of aluminum has been linked to a variety of diseases, including Alzheimer's disease. Aluminum has become more bioavailable since the dawn of the **Aluminum Age** in the 1880's when a process to purify aluminum from bauxite was developed. Like the Stone, Bronze, and Iron Ages that preceded it, the Aluminum Age has brought great changes, both good and bad, to human civilization.

In addition to the factors making life sustainable on earth, as discussed by Henderson in his book, we can now add silicon, the second most abundant element in the earth's crust. In the earth's crust silicon is bonded to oxygen, the most abundant element in the earth's crust, resulting in silica and its fully hydrated form OSA that facilitates the detoxification of aluminum, the third most abundant element in the earth's crust.

I have written three other books:

- "Prevent Alzheimer's, Autism, and Stroke"
- "Increased IQ, Cognition and COVID-19 Cure Rate with Essential Nutrients"
- "Finding a Cause and Potential Cures for Alzheimer's Disease"

There are also five videos on You Tube:

- "Brain Fitness in the Aluminum Age – Preventing Alzheimer's"
- "Brain Fitness in the Aluminum Age - Eliminating Aluminum"
- "Brain Fitness in the Aluminum Age – Coffer Makers"
- "Silica Water – How to Make it at Home"
- "Silica Water for Reversing Alzheimer's

Up to date information is available at my Blog: http://prevent-alzheimers-autism-stroke.blogspot.com/ and my website: http://prevent-alzheimers-autism-stroke.com

In addition, there is information about this book at my Facebook page entitled: "Silica Water the Secret of Healthy Longevity in the Aluminum Age".

Introduction

This book is about **silica water** containing an overlooked miracle molecule that protects our life and maintains our health. It is in our bodies even before birth but during our life it ebbs and flows and needs supplementation to be steadily maintained. This superstar of a molecule is called orthosilicic acid (OSA). For most organisms, including humans, it is essential for life[72]. In fact, it is said that OSA is the most important molecule for life on earth. OSA is a miracle molecule because it protects plants, animals, and even humans from toxic forms of aluminum.

We are fortunate on earth to have oxygen and silicon as the two most abundant elements in the earth's crust. Over millions of years silicon has become oxidized by oxygen to a variety of silicon oxides that have in turn formed into a variety of silicon containing minerals as described in Chapter 1. One of these silicon oxides is OSA, a water-soluble oxide of silicon. As life evolved on earth so did unique ways to use OSA for protection from aluminum, the third most common element in the earth's crust. The mechanisms by which plants and animals, including humans, use OSA as protection from aluminum toxicity are described in Chapter 2.

Aluminum has become more bioavailable since the dawn of the **Aluminum Age** in the 1880's when a process to purify aluminum from bauxite was developed. This has opened a Pandora's Box of aluminum compounds and products that have exponentially increased over the last 120 years and are now in our drinking water, food, kitchen-ware, drugs, vaccines, and even the air we inhale. These products, listed in Appendix II and III, increase both our aluminum ingestion and aluminum accumulation in our bodies. It is chronic aluminum accumulation that is involved in the etiology of a variety of diseases that shorten our lives including: Alzheimer's disease, atherosclerosis (i.e., heart disease), autism, cancer, multiple sclerosis, Parkinson's disease, seizures, and osteoporosis as will be discussed in Chapter 5 of this book.

Writing this book has been a journey, as along the way I have met people who have changed the course of my thinking and writing. For instance, at my local library's author's day I met the author, Martha R.A. Fields, who is originally from Okinawa, Japan. Martha told me that on Okinawa Island there is a high density of centenarians. In addition, demographers have studied Okinawans and found lower than normal rates of Alzheimer's, atherosclerosis, and cancer. They have also found that Okinawans have a higher-than-normal probability of both living to 90+ and being in good health. These facts changed my thinking as Okinawans provide a longitudinal study of what factors are important for avoiding terminal diseases and living a long healthy life.

Drug companies are currently spending millions of dollars on multi-year studies looking for preventatives and cures for Alzheimer's, heart disease, and cancer. What if there are already published studies on populations of 90 to 100-year-olds whose **healthy longevity** is due to abnormally low rates of Alzheimer's, heart disease, and cancer? If these studies exist, they would be equivalent to having century long longitudinal studies just waiting for people to find what they have in common that prevented and possibly cured these diseases.

Amazingly, in addition to Okinawa there are five other small geographic regions on earth that have been identified as having populations with higher survival rates of reaching 90+ years of age than surrounding areas[2]. These geographic regions are called longevity regions in this book in order to not infringe U.S. trademarks. For instance, the word "blue" is part of a commonly used U.S. trademark that describes some of these longevity regions. This is because demographers had circled some of these regions on maps as they were discovered with blue ink[120]. The environment and lifestyle of these longevity regions can potentially teach valuable lessons that may allow us to achieve **healthy longevity** by preventing and possibly healing diseases that can shorten our lives, such as Alzheimer's disease, heart disease, cancer, seizures, multiple sclerosis, and Parkinson's disease.

Could it be that all longevity regions have in common substrata rich in silicate minerals? If so, underground fresh water in contact with substrata could bubble to the surface as OSA rich drinking water. Chapter 3 of this book discloses **the secret of health longevity** - how and why drinking silica rich water results in **healthy longevity**.

By just having silica water (e.g., Fiji water) delivered to their door and eliminating common sources of aluminum from their diet, my parents made their home in Iowa a micro-longevity region. Due to their **resiliency** adapting to changing lifestyles, my mother regained her short-term memory and temporarily stopped the progression of her Alzheimer's disease. My father and mother exemplify what others could do to improve their **individual healthy longevity**.

Chapter 1 – Silica Water

This book is about the type of silica called orthosilicic acid (OSA, a.k.a. reactive silica) as diagrammed in Figure 1. When OSA is dissolved in water the mixture is called silica water.

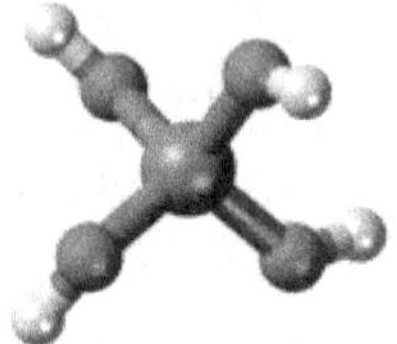

Figure 1 – Orthosilicic acid (OSA)

OSA is soluble in water at low concentrations (e.g., at or below 2 millimolar = mM or 200 parts per million = ppm)[17]. OSA polymerizes above pH 8 at concentrations higher than 200ppm. This polymerization is catalyzed by magnesium and calcium[18,19]. OSA polymerization is also catalyzed at pH 7 by cyanobacteria in contact with ferrihydrite, a commonly found mineral in fresh water and marine environments of the world[20].

Silica water is safe to ingest. It is not an evolutionary accident that dissolved silica is found in mother's breastmilk[21]. Silica water is generally regarded as safe (GRAS) by the U.S. FDA in drinking water at or below 160ppm of OSA ($Si(OH)_4$) or 100ppm of dissolved silica (SiO_2)[22]. OSA is found at low concentrations in most tap water in the U.S.A. OSA is natural occurring and is also added to drinking water by community water companies to control corrosion[23].

There are commercially available natural waters rich in OSA. In the following list the waters tested for OSA concentration are indicated with a "*" (see Appendix I for more silica waters):

- **Starkey Spring Water** from Idaho is available from Whole Foods (93ppm OSA*)
- **Fiji water** from Fiji is available in the U.S.A. (146ppm OSA*)
- **Langkawi Pure** from Malaysia is available in Asia and U.S.A. (133ppm OSA*)
- **Volvic** water from France is available in the U.S.A. and Europe (51 ppm OSA*)
- **Gerolsteiner** from Germany is available in Europe (64ppm OSA*)
- **Acilis** water from Malaysia is available in Europe (88ppm OSA)

As we will see in this book, OSA in drinking water is essential for life and good health leading to greater longevity. OSA supplementation in one's diet is recommended to prevent diseases caused by aluminum. Also, a procedure is described in Chapter 6 for making inexpensive and more sustainable supplementary synthetic OSA from powdered hydrous sodium silicate and sodium bisulfate. This synthetic OSA rich water is called "Silicade" and it contains 146ppm of OSA, identical to Fiji water.

PPM a Unit of Measure of OSA in Silica Water

The weight in milligrams of chemical dissolved in a million milligrams of water is called parts per million or ppm. The ppm unit of measure expresses the concentration of the chemical dissolved in water. The weight per atom of a chemical is called molecular weight (MW). There can be oxygen and hydrogen atoms bonded to elemental silicon forming derivatives of increased MW. The concentration when expressed as "ppm of silicon" must be multiplied by 3.4 to be expressed as "ppm of OSA" because of the additional MW of four OH's. Here are some common conversion factors based upon molecular weight differences:

- Si (MW 28) is called "elemental silicon" that is multiplied by 3.4 to get ppm of OSA
- SiO_2 (MW 60) is called "silica" that is multiplied by 1.6 to get ppm of OSA
- $Si(OH)_4$ (MW 96) is called orthosilicic acid, OSA, or reactive silica

In this book dissolved orthosilicic acid in water is expressed as ppm OSA, unless otherwise specified. Note that one ppm is equivalent to one milligram per liter (a.k.a. 1mg/L)

PPB a Unit of Measure of Aluminum in Water

The weight in milligrams of chemical dissolved in a billion milligrams of water is called parts per billion or ppb. The ppb unit of measure expresses the concentration of the chemical dissolved in water. This is a common unit of measure for aluminum in water. Note that one ppb is equivalent to one microgram per liter (a.k.a. 1mcg/L).

Other Forms of Silicon

Elementary Silicon

Silicon is a chemical element with the symbol Si and it is the second most abundant element in the earth's crust. It is used as a semiconductor for components in electronic products. Silicon has a very high affinity for oxygen that is the most abundant element in the earth's crust. Silicon has been slowly oxidized to silica over millions of years in the earth's oxygen rich environment. Most of the earth's crust is composed of silicon, primarily as silica and silicate containing minerals.

Silicon Dioxide

Silicon dioxide is the anhydride of OSA and is the simplest oxide of silicon with the chemical structure SiO_2. Silicon dioxide is found in nature in many physical forms including:

- Crystalline such as quartz
- Amorphous such as the major component of sand
- Shells of diatoms and radiolariens such as diatomaceous earth
- Colloidal such as commercial silica supplements

These forms of silica have low water solubility and dissolve as OSA very slowly in water on a time-scale of years. Therefore, when they are placed in water, they provide only traces of bioavailable OSA[1]. Also, there are manmade nanometer sized particles (nanoparticles) of silicon dioxide called aerogels and silica gels, such as found in Saguna Colloidal Silicogel. Silicon dioxide in most of these physical forms is considered insoluble, as it takes years to dissolve in water as OSA.

Inhaling fine particles of insoluble silicon dioxide causes irritation and can lead to silicosis, bronchitis, lung cancer, and systemic autoimmune diseases, such as lupus and rheumatoid arthritis[24].

Silica Nanoparticles

Intravenously administered silica nanoparticles cause liver damage in mice[25]. Injection of silica nanoparticles into the body cavity of mice induces an inflammatory response[26]. Some nanoparticles of silicon dioxide have been found to be cytotoxic when tested *in vitro* (i.e., in glass) on three different types of human cells[27].

Orally ingested silica nanoparticles (20nm to 100nm) were determined in a 90-day study of rats to have a no adverse effects limit (NOEAL) of 2,000mg per kilogram per day[28]. No animals were treated over this limit and animals treated at this limit had no treatment-related clinical changes and no histopathological findings were observed in any of the treated animals[28]. Even though inhalation of nanoparticles and injection of nanoparticles into the blood and body cavity should be avoided, the high NOEAL indicates oral ingestion of tenths of a gram of silica nanoparticles a day is safe for rats.

The 2014 finding that oral ingestion of silica nanoparticles is safe for rats is not surprising. Rats and humans eat plants and food derived from plants. Almost all plants make silica nanoparticles, called phytoliths, in an effort to sequester OSA for protection from aluminum toxicity, as discussed later in this chapter. Therefore, rats and humans have evolved to tolerate oral ingestion of phytoliths and even benefit from their consumption. Phytoliths bind tightly with aluminum ions in the gut. This prevents some aluminum from being absorbed by the gut and facilitates the excretion of aluminum as discussed in more detail in Chapter 2.

Silicate Oligomers

Some natural and manmade oligomers (i.e., polymers) of sodium silicate, can be converted to OSA in water at room temperature in a matter of hours at pH 4.7 to a matter of days at pH 7.2[29,30]. In addition, supersaturated OSA in water (e.g., 960ppm) above pH 8 can be converted back to oligomeric colloids of sodium silicate in a matter of hours[29]. These oligomeric colloids are in a pH dependent equilibrium with OSA above OSA's saturation level (i.e., greater than 200ppm) in water. Therefore, these manmade oligomeric colloids of sodium silicate could provide a healthy oral source of less than 200ppm of OSA, only when allowed enough time to dissolve in a sufficient volume of weakly acidic water before oral ingestion.

Natural or manmade oligomers of sodium silicate should not be taken orally without drinking a volume of water sufficient to dissolve and dilute them to below the saturation level of OSA in water (i.e., 200ppm). When this lack of sufficient water occurs, there may be a risk that OSA will crystallize out of a supersaturated OSA solution in the kidneys forming painful silica stones. However, silica kidney stones have never been reported after ingesting oligomers of sodium silicate.

Magnesium Trisilicate

Silica kidney stones do rarely occur in those who ingest large amounts of magnesium trisilicate without drinking a sufficient volume of water[31]. Magnesium trisilicate is a compound of silicon dioxide (not less than 45%) and magnesium oxide (not less than 20%) the rest being water. Magnesium trisilicate is used in some antacids as it reacts to neutralize stomach acid. It is also used by fast food chains, such as KFC, to absorb fatty acids and remove impurities that form in the edible oils during the frying process.

Unlike sodium silicate that is soluble in water (22.2gr./100cc), magnesium trisilicate is practically insoluble in water. Ingesting undissolved silicates is a health risk because without adequate water intake the silicates can become supersaturated in the kidney lumen and polymerize or crystallize forming stones (a.k.a. silica uroliths) containing primarily silica (a.k.a. silica urolithiasis). In general silicon containing kidney stones are rare and only found in those who consume large amounts of magnesium trisilicate[31].

Silicones

Silicones (a.k.a. polysiloxanes) are manmade polymers of siloxane ($[Si\text{-}O]_n$) usually with carbon and/or hydrogen atoms bonded to the silicon atom. These polymers are very stable and used for grease, rubber, resin, and lubricants. Silicones are also used for cooking utensils and coatings on cookware. These applications of silicones are considered safe.

Gels of silicones are used for breast implants. If the implant ruptures, silicone leaking from the implant can cause inflammatory nodules in the breast and armpit areas and enlarged lymph glands in the armpit areas of the body[32].

Chapter 2 – Silica Water for Protection from Aluminum

Silica Water is Essential for Diatoms and Radiolarians

The old adage that good things come in small packages is definitely true for some microscopic life forms that use polymerized silicon dioxide for their elaborate skeletons. Examples of these primitive life forms are diatoms and radiolarians. Their skeletons are almost pure silica and appear to be elaborate, delicate, and breathtakingly beautiful baskets that protect these simple organisms as shown in Figure 2.

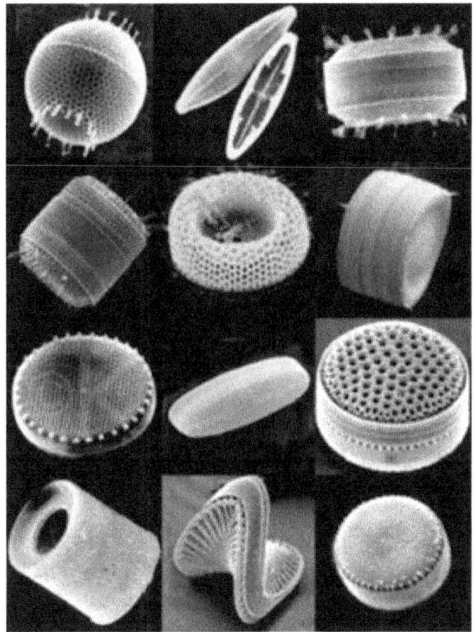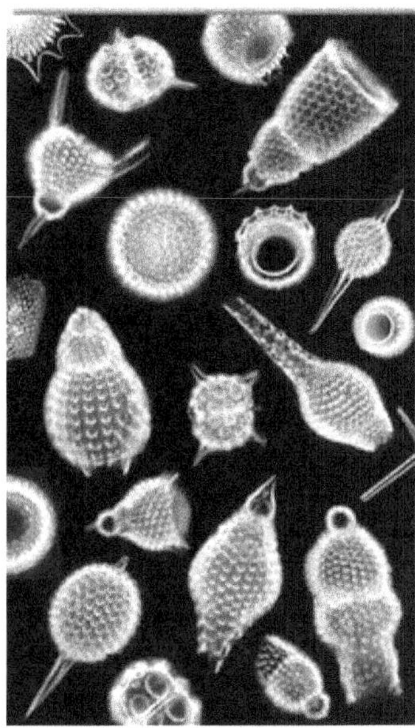

Figure 2 – Diatom Skeletons on the Left and Radiolarian Skeletons on the Right

Diatoms and radiolarians are unicellular microalgae that are plentiful in the oceans of the world accounting for 40% of global oceanic biological productivity[33]. This level of productivity requires a stable concentration of OSA in ocean water. When these organisms die, the silica in their skeletons very slowly dissolves helping to keep the oceanic concentration of OSA constant at 2ppm near the surface. Other sources of silica are slowly dissolving chert, clay, silt, and sand as terrestrial detritus carried by rivers into the oceans.

Radiolarians evolved approximately 542 million years ago in the Paleozoic Era. Diatoms are the new kids on the block having tremendous evolutionary success beginning in the late Mesozoic Era and exponentially increasing in the Eocene Epoch (a.k.a. first half of the Cenozoic Era) around 56 to 34 million years ago. Diatoms currently account for 90 percent of the suspended silica in the oceans. Vast amounts of undissolved diatoms and radiolarians have settled to the bottom of the world's oceans. Over millions of years some of these ocean sediments have become uplifted and made a part of regional subsurface geology. Some limestone and chert containing formations have high amounts of silica due to fossilized skeletons of diatoms and radiolarians. Regions of the world with these formations are more likely to have high levels of OSA in drinking and irrigation water. Examples include:

- Naha Limestone that underlies Okinawa Island[14,15]
- Sedimentary Late Mesozoic to Eocene Limestone that underlies Villagrande, Sardinia[10,34]
- Chert in Punta Conchal Formation that underlies Nicoya, Costa Rica.[35]

The high levels of OSA in the drinking and irrigation water of the Okinawan, Sardinian, and Nicoyan longevity regions is likely due to these subsurface diatomaceous and radiolarian deposits.

How Silica Water Provides Protection from Aluminum

Aluminum in any one of a number of chemical forms is toxic to both plants and animals[43,59]. In acidic water, below pH 4.5, aluminum is ionic having three positive charges. Nearer neutrality, in water above pH 5.5, ionic aluminum is hydroxylated with OH^- ions from water molecules to make monomeric and dimeric aluminum hydroxide[36]. In this case monomers are single molecules of aluminum hydroxide and dimers are two molecules of aluminum hydroxide condensed together as shown in Figure 3[37]. Both the hydroxylations and the condensation are reversible in acidic water below pH 4.5[38].

Dissolved silica (i.e., OSA) detoxifies aluminum. Silicon and aluminum have some similarities as they are next to each other on the periodic table of elements and they both have an affinity for oxygen. OSA, and the dimer of aluminum hydroxide are a match made in heaven. Depending on the ratio of dissolved silica to aluminum in water, one or two molecules of OSA condense above pH 5.5 with a dimer of aluminum hydroxide to form one of the two stable hydroxyaluminosilicate (HAS) complexes HAS_A and HAS_B diagramed in Figure 3[37].

- HAS_A is a stable 1 to 1 complex of OSA and aluminum hydroxide dimer that forms when there is less than a 1 to 1 ratio of OSA to aluminum in water[39,40].
- HAS_B is a stable 2 to 1 complex of OSA and aluminum hydroxide dimer that forms when there is at least a 1 to 1 ratio of OSA to aluminum in water[39,40].

Both of these complexes are non-toxic. Below pH 4.5 these relatively insoluble crystalline complexes are slowly hydrolyzed back into OSA and toxic ionic aluminum[40].

Plants and animals have evolved to use OSA for protection from aluminum. Plants store sequestered aluminum as HAS_B in both apoplasts and biosilifications, such as phytoliths. While animals both store sequestered aluminum as HAS_A in lysosomes and excrete aluminum as dilute HAS_B back into the environment in urine and perspiration. These schemes make use of the chemistry of OSA and aluminum to provide protection from toxic aluminum in the environment. These schemes have worked for millions of years but with the advent of the aluminum age some have proven to be insufficient to handle the recently introduced higher levels of aluminum.

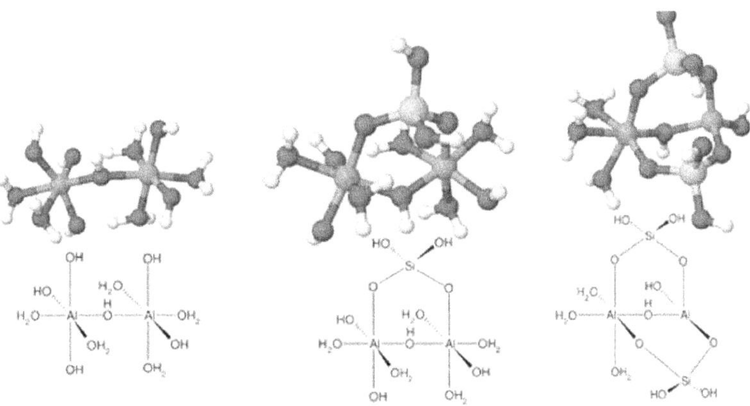

Figure 3 – Aluminum hydroxide dimer on the left, HAS_A in the middle and HAS_B on the right[37]

Silica Water Protects Plants

In the hilly woods near where I live there is a flat tennis court sized area that for as long as anyone can remember has been devoid of all but sparse grass. Trees and a natural berm on one side of this area shield it from view by anyone on the nearest street. A lack of plants over a few inches high indicates a lack of root growth in this area. Why is this small area devoid of plants taller than a few inches?

Finding a clue involves only digging a hole a few inches deep to reveal a thin layer of clay. The local oral history of this unique place involves going back to the 1930's when the preacher of the local First Congregational Church told his flock to not perform recreational sports on Sundays in favor of prayer and bible reading. In order to avoid the preacher's wrath some sports-minded members of his flock surreptitiously built a natural clay tennis court out of his watchful eye. It must have been popular because rumor has it that even the preacher's wife could be found on some Sunday afternoons at the tennis court in the woods.

Some theorize that clay blocking water from reaching roots is the reason for no tall plants. But actually, the reason is soil chemistry. Natural clay used for the tennis court in the woods consists of an aluminum containing mineral called kaolinite. Aluminum is released from kaolinite as aluminum ions when acid rain below pH 4.5 falls on the natural clay[41,42]. Aluminum ions are phytotoxic to root growth as shown in Figure 4[43]. In fact, aluminum phytotoxicity in acid soils is one of the biggest limitations to worldwide crop production[44].

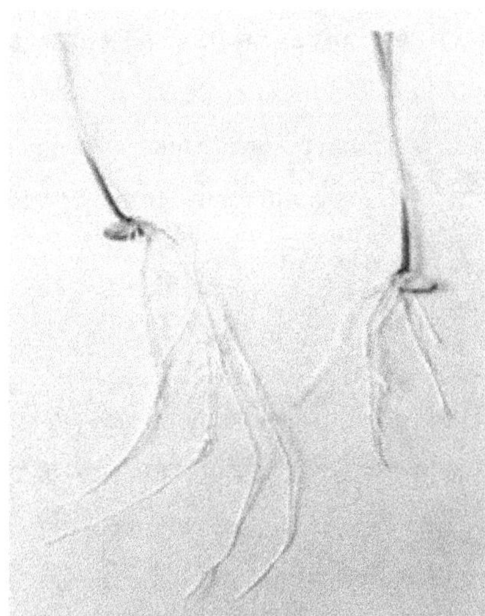

Figure 4 – The effect of low (left) and high (right) aluminum levels on root growth of grasses[43]

Although silicon is not considered essential for plants, plants have evolved incredible ways to use OSA and silica for protection from phytotoxic aluminum. Seven of the ten most important crops in the world are silicon accumulators with above 1% of these plants by dry weight being silicon[44]. It is generally agreed that plants accumulate silica by absorbing OSA either actively or passively from the soil or airborne aerosols. OSA has been found to protect the roots of the following plants from aluminum phytotoxicity: maize (a.k.a. corn)[45], barley[46], soybean[47], and sorghum[48].

In the case of maize (*Zea mays*) the mechanism by which aluminum inhibits root growth has been studied[49]. Aluminum slowly diffuses through the outer epidermal layers of roots cells accumulating in the growing root tip. This causes the plant to respond by producing a plant polysaccharide called callose in the epidermis of the root tip. Callose catalyzes the polymerization of sub-saturated OSA forming insoluble silica in the epidermal cells of the root tip[49,50]. This silica becomes a rigid barrier to aluminum diffusion as the silica binds tightly to aluminum[30]. It is theorized that this rigidification of the epidermal layers of the root tip in response to aluminum results in inhibition of root growth[49].

In addition, cells in the roots of maize actively accumulate OSA in their apoplast[45]. The apoplast is the space inside the cell wall but outside the root cell's plasma membrane where chemicals can diffuse freely though a continuum of adjacent cell walls. Nutrients and toxins use the apoplastic route in order to gain entry through the plasma membrane into a root cell. OSA sequestered in the apoplast complexes with phytotoxic aluminum forming non-phytotoxic HAS (hydroxyaluminosilicates) preventing aluminum from entering root cells and protecting the plant[45].

Trees also absorb OSA and an example is Norway Spruce (*Picea abies*). This absorbed OSA was found to ameliorate the phytotoxic effects of aluminum on Norway Spruce seedlings grown hydroponically above pH 4.5[51]. How is this protection possible as this is below pH 5.5 needed for HAS formation? The explanation is OSA detoxifies aluminum to form HAS only inside root cells of the Norway Spruce seedlings where the pH is actively increased from 4.5 outside to 5.5 inside the root cells. This pH increase is performed by root cells actively absorbing and accumulating OSA from the hydroponic solution[52].

Another way plants detoxify aluminum is sequestration in solid silica phytoliths (a.k.a. biogenic opal) made of polymerized OSA. The word phytoliths is Greek for plant stones. Phytoliths are microscopic structures made of silica by the plant and shown in Figure 5. After plants die, the phytoliths become fossils that can last for millions of years. Because carbon becomes occluded in some phytoliths they can be radiocarbon-dated. The phytoliths in Figure 5 are 9,000 years old and were made by rice plants in China at the beginning of the Holocene Period[53].

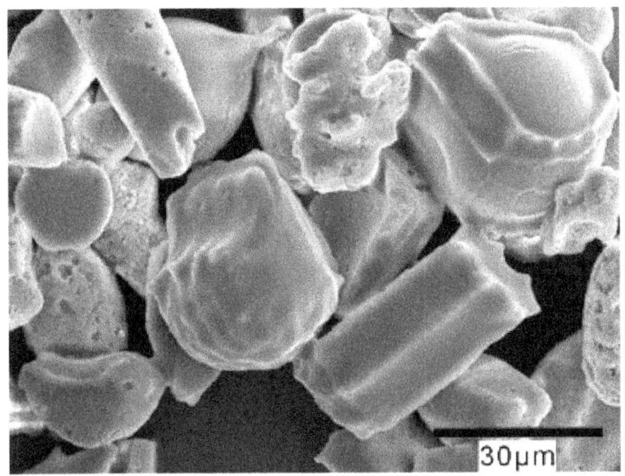

Figure 5 – Scanning electron micrograph of rice phytoliths[53]

The sequestration of sub-saturated OSA in water at less than 200ppm by conversion into solid silica structures, such as phytoliths, in plants is called biosilicification. As in the case of maize, this conversion is catalyzed by callose made by plants in response to injury, including aluminum toxicity[50,54]. The resulting structures are biosilicified mirror images of the cellular and subcellular parts of the plant on which they are deposited. When looked at in a microscope, after staining for silica, the structures look breathtakingly beautiful. An example is the picture of three biosilicified stomata on a distal stem of horsetail as shown in Figure 6[50].

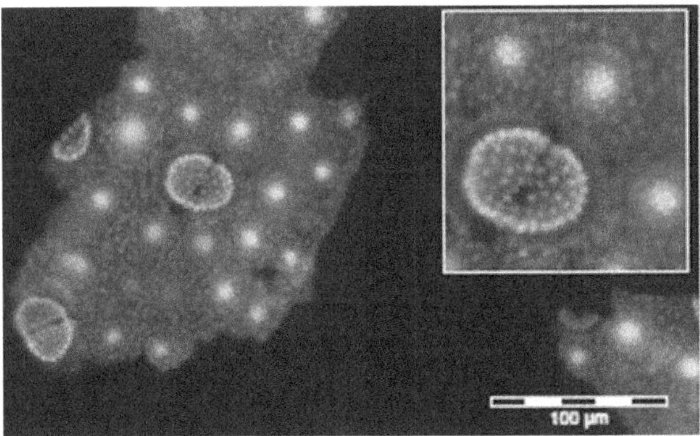

Figure 6 – Fluorescent stained heavily biosilicified stomata on distal stem of horsetail[50]

Biosilifications - an Aluminum Filter for Air-Plants

The stomata of plants are small ports through which plants breathe by transpiring oxygen, carbon dioxide, and water vapor and by reverse-transpiring water vapor and liquid hygroscopic aerosols that collect on plant leaves[55]. Hydraulic activation of stomata allows bidirectional liquid aerosol transport between leaf surface and leaf interior[56]. Aerosols have always been a component of the earth's atmosphere and plant surfaces are a major aerosol sink. Aerosols that have collected on leaves can contain nutrients, such as OSA, that are transferred through the stomata to the interior of the leaves[56]. Also, aerosols can contain phytotoxic chemicals, such as aluminum.

The stomata in some plants, such as the bird's-nest fern (*Asplenium nidus*), are rich in callose and as a result become sites for silica deposition[50,57]. Polymeric OSA has a high affinity for aluminum[30] and when deposited as insoluble silica around the stomata of plants it makes every stoma an aluminum filter (see Figure 6). This is useful for the bird's-nest fern as it is an air-plant (a.k.a. epiphyte) growing on another plant, such as a tree but not deriving sustenance from the tree. When the bird's nest fern collects airborne nutrient containing aerosols on its leaves, it uses deposited silica to filter any aluminum before it is transferred through the stomata into the leaf.

Phytoliths from the wood and leaves of sub-alpine plant species were found in 72% of the cases to contain a significant percentage of hydroxyaluminosilicate[58]. This underscores the commonality of plants using OSA and biosilifications for aluminum detoxification.

Plants have evolved to protect themselves from phytotoxic aluminum by detoxifying and sequestering aluminum in apoplasts and biosilifications, such as phytoliths. This only works in areas where there is available OSA in the soil. In some areas of the world with OSA deficient soil, OSA is currently used as a fertilizer to ultimately provide plants with protection from phytotoxic aluminum[44].

Silica Water Protects Animals

I am an avid fisherman and love catching and releasing trout. Some years ago I spotted a small remote pond from a mountain top in New Hampshire. After some hiking and route finding, involving map and compass, I arrived at the pond but there appeared to be no trout in the pond. Remarkably there was a limnologist studying this pond. After surprisingly appearing out of the brush along the edge of the pond, he pointed out that there were no trout in this pond due to acid rain. The acid rain had liberated a toxin out of the rock and soil around the pond and this toxin had killed the fish and other aquatic life in the pond. By his analysis of the pond's water, aluminum ions were the toxin.

Aluminum ions in water at a concentration of 350ppb and a pH of 5.5 kills fish in 48 hours by damaging their gills and preventing the fish from getting oxygen from water[59]. In 1989 it was reported by Birchall et al. that OSA detoxifies 350ppb of aluminum. To prove this OSA at twice the concentration of aluminum in water (2mM OSA and 1mM aluminum) was diluted 77-fold resulting in a solution that contained 350ppb of aluminum and 2.5ppm of OSA. This solution did not kill fish at pH 5.5[59]. Exley, et al., also proved that HAS_B formed at pH 5.5 under these same conditions was nontoxic to fish[60]. This work demonstrated that OSA can passively protect fish in water polluted with aluminum.

The lives of animals are both passively and actively protected from aluminum toxicity by OSA. Animals on earth have evolved the ability to actively accumulate OSA in order to protect them from aluminum poisoning. This evolution started millions of years ago in primitive animals, such as snails. Snails (*Lymnaea stagnalis*), when exposed to 555ppb of aluminum and 0.158ppm of OSA in water, increase their level of OSA in intracellular organelles, called lysosomes, as compared with snails not exposed to aluminum. This results in aluminum detoxification by sequestration in lysosomal granules of digestive cells in the digestive gland of snails[61].

The ratio of silicon to aluminum is 1:2.3 in snail lysosomes indicating that the aluminum has been detoxified to HAS_A[61]. Since the level of OSA in the snail's water is too low for HAS_A to form prior to entry into the lysosome, snails actively increase the OSA level in their lysosomes to a level sufficient to form HAS_A in response to aluminum in their water.

In higher animals, such as rats, Carlisle and Curran at UCLA School of Public Health found that when rats were fed a supplemental aluminum with low OSA diet, 23-month-old rats had not accumulated aluminum in their brains, while 28-month rats had accumulated aluminum in their brains. Both 23-month-old and 28-month-old rats fed a supplemental aluminum with high OSA diet, did not accumulate aluminum in their brains[62]. This observation is indicative of OSA either facilitating the excretion of aluminum or impairing the sequestration of aluminum in the aging rat brain. They concluded[62]:

"Dietary silicon supplementation thus appeared to be protective against aluminum accumulation in an ageing brain."

In an effort to confirm Carlisle and Curran's findings, supplemental aluminum, as aluminum nitrate, was given to young rats (21 days old), adult rats (8 months old), and old rats (16 months old). The aluminum was administered by gavage (i.e., through a tube to the stomach) daily for 6.5 months and then the animal's brains were analyzed for aluminum accumulation. Contrary to Carlisle and Curran's findings, rats of all ages accumulated aluminum in their brains[63]. The olfactory bulb of the brain had the highest aluminum levels.

In an effort to find if accumulated aluminum as found in the organs of rats decreased with OSA supplementation, rats were simultaneously given both supplemental OSA and aluminum. Patterning OSA dosages after Carlisle and Curran[62], supplemental synthetic OSA was given to rats for 5 weeks and concurrently supplemental aluminum was given by gavage for just 5 days a week for 5 weeks[64]. This OSA treatment decreases both the prior accumulated aluminum, as measured in the control animals, and ingested supplemental aluminum in four organs and six regions of the brain[64]. Table 1 summarizes this important, remarkable, and disturbing data.

The most important point of Table 1 is comparing the control data, representing aluminum accumulated prior the start of the experiment (column 2), and the amounts of aluminum remaining after supplementation with 200 and 400ppm OSA (columns 4 and 5). **Note after OSA supplementation the accumulated aluminum is reduced in all organs and regions of the brain even in spite of aluminum supplementation!** This result shows the power of OSA to purge the body of accumulated aluminum in a matter of weeks.

Importance:

- In every tissue and organ tested, including bone and six regions of brain, the prior accumulated aluminum is reversed by supplemental OSA.
- Aluminum accumulation is possibly an adverse effect of aging.
- Both rats and humans are mammals and what happens in rats is usually also true for humans.

Remarkable:

- The reversal in aluminum accumulation is dose dependent averaging 58% with 200ppm of OSA and 79% with 400ppm of supplemental OSA.
- OSA at twice its saturation level in water (i.e., 400ppm) is more effective at lowering aluminum accumulation than at its 200ppm saturation level. This implies that insoluble OSA oligomers (i.e., short polymers), formed in supersaturated OSA, may bind to some of the supplemental aluminum in the gut preventing aluminum absorption[30].
- There is less aluminum in urine with 200ppm OSA supplementation than without 200ppm OSA supplementation. Therefore, because OSA at 200ppm does not form oligomers, OSA monomers must also bind to some of the supplemental aluminum in the gut preventing aluminum absorption[64].

Disturbing:

- Aluminum accumulation in young rats indicates that early stages of the life cycle allow aluminum accumulation in the brain, such as seen in children with autism who accumulate more aluminum in their brains than children without autism[63,65].
- Highest aluminum accumulation in the olfactory bulb suggests aluminum nitrate in water was inhaled during or immediately after gavage. This may be a preferred route of entry into the brain, possibly because it is a shortcut that avoids the blood-brain-barrier[66-69].

Table 1. Reversing Aluminum (Al) Accumulation with OSA Supplementation[64]				
Organ / Tissue	Al in Control	Al with: no OSA	200ppm OSA	400ppm OSA
Supplemental	Al = No	= Yes	= Yes	= Yes
Liver	0.78 ± 0.69	4.39 ± 1.56	0.14 ± 0.38	0.96 ± 0.14
Bone	8.95 ± 2.90	16.30 ± 4.95	4.54 ± 1.15	1.46 ± 0.61
Spleen	3.24 ± 3.89	6.77 ± 2.03	0.29 ± 0.40	0.46 ± 0.57
Kidney	1.38 ± 1.31	3.33 ± 3.05	1.24 ± 0.48	0.45 ± 0.51
Brain:				
Cortex	3.98 ± 3.38	57.18 ± 18.87	1.56 ± 2.60	1.09 ± 0.91
Hippocampus	2.41 ± 4.33	17.08 ± 10.34	ND	1.32 ± 1.07
Striatum	7.12 ± 5.18	15.82 ± 8.59	1.93 ± 3.84	1.16 ± 1.41
Cerebellum	11.01 ± 5.39	62.13 ± 11.69	12.02 ± 2.36	2.01 ± 2.36
Thalamus	7.25 ± 7.88	41.58 ± 35.22	2.06 ± 4.95	0.74 ± 0.43
Olfactory Bulb	36.94 ± 35.34	124.30 ± 109.78	24.59 ± 20.01	0.96 ± 1.93

Results are micrograms of aluminum per gram wet weight of organ or tissue. ND = not detected, Detection limit 0.001micrograms/gr.

A certain minimal dose of OSA in water administered over a sufficient period of time is required to increase the elimination of aluminum and lower aluminum absorption in rats and humans. For instance, Volvic water (51 ppm OSA) was given as drinking water to rats for one week. At the 5-day point both aluminum-26 (i.e., a radioactive isotope of aluminum) and 0.2cc of Volvic water were given to the rats by gavage. In this experiment OSA did not increase aluminum-26 elimination in the urine or lower aluminum-26 accumulation in the bones of rats[70]. Likewise, only 1 dose of 0.6 liters of synthetic 187ppm OSA given to 5 human volunteers resulted in increased aluminum excretion occurring simultaneously with peak silica excretion but at a level too small to be significant[71]. **These results suggest that when silica water is administered in too low a volume or for too short a time, there will be no observable benefit.** In contrast it has been observed that 1.5 liters of Volvic water drunk within 1 hour is sufficient to enhance aluminum elimination in humans as described it the next section of this chapter.

Independent of OSA's ability to protect animals from aluminum toxicity, the essentiality of silicon in animals has been established by a series of experiments[72]:

- Silicon was shown to be localized in bone growth areas of young mice and rats
- Silicon is required for normal growth and skeletal development in chicks
- Silicon is required for bone growth and skull formation in rats

Animal protection from toxic aluminum by OSA is both passive and active. Snails actively sequester OSA for aluminum protection. Fish passively derive gill protection from OSA in water. Rats passively benefit from OSA and OSA oligomers in drinking water that bind with aluminum in the gut, preventing absorption, and facilitating aluminum excretion in feces and urine. Rats may actively transport OSA to the kidney lumen and urine in order to prevent aluminum reabsorption into the blood. Aluminum stores in organs and tissues are in a dynamic equilibrium. Supplemental OSA dramatically shifts this equilibrium in favor of aluminum elimination from organs and tissues and into the urine for excretion.

It is now generally accepted that silicon, as OSA, is an essential nutritional trace element for animals[72]. But until recently the essentiality for humans had not been established. In humans, loss of silicon with ageing is linked to loss of tissue flexibility[72]:

- Silicon content of the human aorta and other arterial vessels declines with age leading to less flexibility
- Silicon content of the human arterial wall declines in parallel with atherosclerosis (a.k.a. hardening of the arteries)
- Silicon content of skin declines leading to wrinkling

Over millions of years plant and animals have evolved protective mechanisms using OSA to actively and passively protect themselves from aluminum toxicity. But with arrival of the aluminum age these protective mechanisms have become insufficient to handle the increasing levels of aluminum in the environment. As an example, humans are susceptible to mismatch diseases in which our body's evolved defenses for aluminum are not up to the task of protecting us. This results in mismatch diseases such as Alzheimer's, autism, cardiovascular disease (i.e., chronic heart disease and stroke), Parkinson's, and multiple sclerosis.

Also, in humans declining blood OSA levels with ageing may be linked to an increase in aluminum absorption in the old and elderly. The essentiality of OSA for active aluminum protection for humans is addressed in the next section of Chapter 2.

Silica Water Protects Humans

In humans the complexation of OSA with aluminum hydroxide dimer to form HAS_B can occur in the duodenum (pH 5.8-6.7), blood (pH 7.4), kidney lumen, (pH 6.5 to 8.0), and across the blood-brain-barrier in the cerebrospinal fluid (pH 7.33). In addition, it has been shown in a human test that at least 3.6% of ingested OSA goes inside cells within 2 hours of ingestion and has an intracellular half-life of 11 hours[481]. During this time complexation of OSA with aluminum can occur inside human cells that are normally at pH 6.8 to 7.4. The formation of HAS_B protects humans from aluminum toxicity by facilitating the excretion of aluminum in urine, feces, and perspiration[73,74]. It has been shown that a diet that includes a mineral water high in OSA facilitates both the urination and perspiration pathways for aluminum excretion[75].

The best way to measure the effect of OSA on aluminum excretion is to feed humans radioactive ionic aluminum-26 with and without OSA supplementation and follow its level in blood plasma and urine over a period of time. This test is risky for volunteers who participate, as aluminum-26 decays so energetically that its recommend storage is in a chamber lined with 2 inches of lead[76]. In spite of this danger, J. A. Edwardson in 1993 found that OSA (100uM/L = 96ppm) in orange juice laced with isotopic aluminum-26 lowers human blood plasma levels by 10-fold on average compared with the same human volunteers drinking aluminum-26 laced orange juice without OSA[77]. This data is on the left in Figure 7. In order to measure how quickly absorbed aluminum is excreted in the urine, a healthy volunteer's aluminum level in urine was measured hourly after drinking 1.5 liters of 51ppm OSA in Volvic water[78]. This data is on the right in Figure 7.

Silica water enriched with OSA can be made synthetically by diluting and acidifying sodium silicate and purchased as either silica rich bottled drinking water or beer with and without alcohol. All of these sources of OSA have been tested for their ability to enhance aluminum excretion by measuring aluminum-26 or aluminum-28 in blood plasma or urine as summarized in Table 2. Ingesting synthetic or natural OSA demonstrates that in both cases there is similar bioavailability of OSA[30,79,80]. Also in both cases after drinking OSA rich water the amount of aluminum in the blood and excreted in the urine reaches a maximum after several hours and then declines (see Figure 7)[77,78].

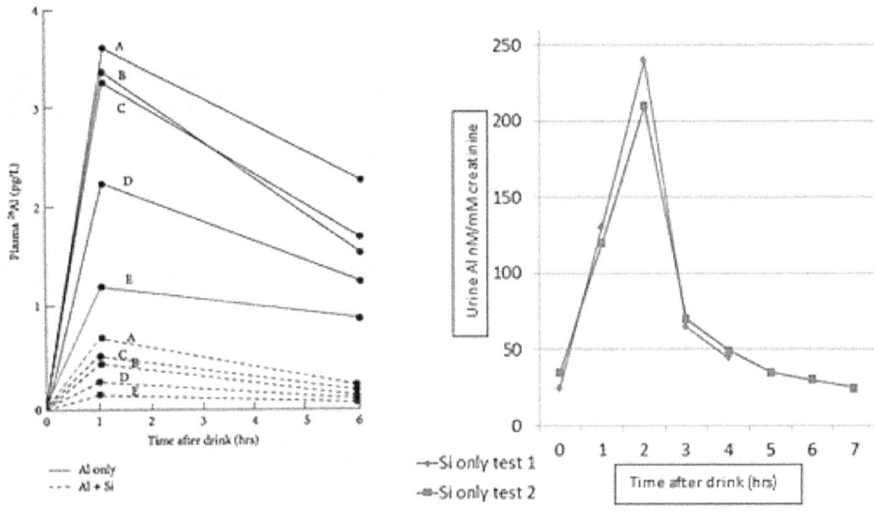

Figure 7 – Effect of OSA on aluminum in blood plasma and urine[77,78]

Left Graph – Aluminum-26 levels in blood: Five healthy volunteers (A-E) first drank orange juice containing aluminum-26 without OSA and (solid lines) then several days later drank the same aluminum-26 laced orange juice with OSA (dashed lines)[77]. **Right Graph – Aluminum divided by creatinine levels in urine:** One healthy volunteer drank 1.5 liters of OSA (51ppm) and then repeated the test approx. 1 week later by drinking another 1.5 liters of OSA (51ppm) [78].

Table 2. Natural and Synthetic OSA Enhances Urinary Aluminum (Al) Excretion						
Source of OSA	Number of Volunteers	OSA (ppm)	% Bioavailability OSA	Dose (Liters)	% Enhancement of Al excretion	Ref.
Synthetic						
Silicate	3	96	53.2 ± 8.5	0.6	75*	30
Silicate	5	111	43.1 ± 8	0.66	ND	79
Natural						
Spritzer	14	119	ND	1.0/day	60*	73
Beer**	6	64	56 ± 8	1.13	125*	80
Beer***	5	118	60.1 ± 3	0.66	ND	79

* Urinary excretion   ** Alcoholic beer   *** Alcohol free beer   ND = Not determined

The date in Table 2 is consistent with OSA facilitating an enhanced excretion of accumulated aluminum in the urine[80].   Enhanced urinary excretion of aluminum occurs within hours of ingesting OSA. With continued ingestion of OSA over three months, accumulated aluminum is significantly decreased in the body[73]. **The data in Table 2 proves that the source of OSA, be it either synthetic, such as silicate, or natural, such as Spritzer or beer, does not matter as OSA from all these sources enhances aluminum excretion.**

The duodenum is the primary site of aluminum absorption in the gastrointestinal tract of rats and humans[81]. Human duodenal pH is 5.8 to 6.5 during fasting and 6.0 to 6.7 while eating and the kidney lumen is pH 6.5 to 8.0.[82]. Therefore, OSA can react with aluminum hydroxide dimer in both the duodenum and the kidney lumen to form HAS_B and thereby prevent both aluminum and OSA from being absorbed from the duodenum into the blood and reabsorbed from the urine into blood. From the data in the plot on the left side of Figure 7, some humans given supplemental OSA excrete 3 times more aluminum than others[77]. This indicates the possibility of active OSA sequestration in the kidney lumen that varies among individuals.

OSA also facilitates the excretion of aluminum in human perspiration[74]. Before drinking OSA rich water males and females age 20-22 who are exercising excrete the same concentration of aluminum in sweat as shown in Table 3[74]. After drinking OSA rich water both males and females excrete 1.5 to 2.4 fold higher levels of aluminum than before drinking OSA rich water as shown in Table 3[74]. However, males excrete more aluminum than females because males at age 18-24 have greater sweat gland output than females[83,84]. Note that the volume of sweat per day (e.g., 3 to 4 liters an hour while exercising) can exceed the volume of urine per day (i.e., less than 2 liters/day).

Table 3. OSA Facilitates Aluminum Excretion in Human Perspiration[74]					
		Before Drinking OSA		**After Drinking OSA**	
Subjects	**# of Subjects**	**Al in Sweat avg. mcg/L**	**Si in Sweat avg. mcg/L**	**Al in Sweat avg. mcg/L**	**Si in Sweat avg. mcg/L**
Males	9	340	830	1200	1770
Females	10	350	680	840	1560

Kristien Van Dyke in 2000 measured the OSA content of blood serum in different aged individuals[85]. Dr. Van Dyke found very high levels of OSA in infants less than a year old and extremely low levels in pregnant mothers. This data is diagrammed in Figure 8. Dr. Van Dyke came to a startling conclusion:

"The explanation of the high silicon levels of the infant group, especially <1yr., may be that pregnant mothers offer their silicon to the growing fetus …"

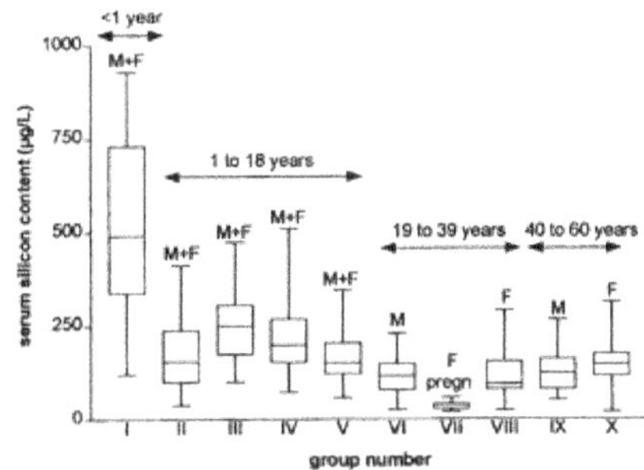

Figure 8 – Box plot of serum silicon content of various groups
(M: male; F: female; pregn: pregnant women)[85]

The soluble silicon in the blood serum is OSA and there is also OSA in breastmilk. Tanaka in 1990 found levels of silicon in breastmilk of 470 to 670mcg/liter from 1 week to 1 month of birth[21]. These findings suggest that OSA is a nutrient that mothers have evolved to supply to the fetus and infant. OSA not only lowers levels of absorbed aluminum in the brain[62,64] but also improves bone mineral density and strength[86-88].

Conclusion of Silica Water for Protection from Aluminum

It is amazing that plants, animals, and humans all use OSA, a naturally occurring molecule, to provide protection from aluminum toxicity. It is equally amazing that mother's give their OSA to their fetuses and infants to provide protection from aluminum. This discovery elevates the importance of OSA to that of an essential nutrient in humans[85]. **In conclusion from the very simple life forms, such as diatoms and radiolarians, to very complex organisms, such as humans, OSA has been found to play essential roles.**

Chapter 3 – Silica Water for Healthy Longevity

"If there is magic on this planet, it is contained in the water."

Loren C. Eiseley – The Immense Journey 1946

In my first book on preventing Alzheimer's disease and atherosclerosis by using OSA in drinking water to lower chronic aluminum toxicity there was no mention that this could also result in increased longevity[1]. However, these diseases do shorten the lives of a large percentage of the worldwide population. But does drinking OSA rich silica water actually increase longevity?

This question was on my mind when I met the author Martha R. A. Fields at the local library sponsored author's day. Martha was originally from Okinawa and explained that Okinawans live longer than Japanese and much longer than those in the U.S.A. She was most fascinated with the fact that Okinawans have an ikigai (pronounced "ick-ee-guy") that means a reason for being. This more purposeful approach to work and life is believed to result in longevity. I became fascinated when she mentioned that extensive research had been conducted on Okinawans. My detective instincts started my journey as I wondered if in general do Okinawans both have an ikigai and drink OSA rich silica water.

There are hot spots of longevity on earth that have been identified by demographers who carefully checked through birth and death records. These geographic regions are called longevity regions in this book. Demographers circled at least one of these geographic regions with blue ink on a map and for this reason they called it a blue region[120]. In these regions, when compared with surrounding regions, there are higher concentrations of 100-year-olds (centenarians) and higher probability of 60-79-year-olds in 1970 surviving to 90+ by year 2000 (see Table 3)[2]. The people of these regions have less dementia, heart disease, certain cancers, and osteoporosis accounting for their longevity.

By 2022 six longevity regions have been identified:

- **Okinawa, Japan** – The largest island in a subtropical archipelago that has the world's longest-lived women.
- **Villagrande, Sardinia** – A small mountainous region on an island off the coast of Italy with the world's highest concentration of male centenarians.
- **Ikaria, Greece** – An island off the coast of Greece in the Aegean Sea that has one of the lowest rates of middle age mortality in the world and the lowest rate of dementia in the world.
- **Nicoya Peninsula, Costa Rica** – A region where residents have one of lowest rates of middle age mortality in the world and the second highest concentration of male centenarians.
- **Loma Linda, California** – City with the highest concentration of Seventh-day Adventists in the U.S.A. where they live ten years longer than the average American.
- **Western Hechi, China** – A three county area with much higher centenarian density and more than double the likelihood of reaching 90 years of age than three boarding counties to the east.

In Table 4 the male and female survival rates are the percentage of people 60 to 79 who will make it to age 90 in each country and longevity region. The longevity index is the percentage of people 65 to 89 who will make it to age 90. This table shows that either male and female survival rates or the longevity index is higher in longevity regions than each of their nearby areas. The table also shows that all longevity regions sit either atop or near silica rich substrates that results in silica rich water used for both drinking and crop irrigation. The longevity regions provide us with clues as to why people who live there live longer. Higher than normal levels of silica in drinking water are more than a clue; they are a loud and clear message that silica water can prevent and heal diseases that shorten our lives, such as Alzheimer's, cardiovascular disease (e.g., heart disease and stroke), some cancers, osteoporosis, and multiple sclerosis.

Table 4 – Longevity Regions and OSA in Drinking Water				
Country & Longevity Region	1970-2000 Male Survival Rate[2]	1970-2000 Female Survival Rate[2]	Drinking Water Source	OSA ppm
Japan-Honshu	3.5	10.5	Tap Water	26[12,13]
Okinawa	6.6	16.3	Northern Rivers & Res.	40[14-16]
Italy	2.0	6.1	Bottled Mineral Water	17[8]
Sardinia	3.9	6.7	Thermal Springs	15–69[9,10]
Villagrande	8.9	8.6	Thermal Springs	24–67[11]
Greece	1.7	4.2	Rivers & Reservoirs	13***[142]
Ikaria	2.5	5.7	Thermal Springs	18–58[7]
Costa Rica	8.0	10.7	Rivers Near Tiribi Tuff*	28-45[154]
Nicoya	9.4	11.2	Tempisque River Basin[6]	59–141[6]
USA	2.9	7.7	Tap Water	11[3]
Loma Linda	?	?	Bunker Hill Basin[4,5]	32.5[5]
Adventists	?	?	48-64 oz./day of water	65**
Hechi, China	2000 Longevity Index (90+/65+)[461]			
Central Hechi	1.6****		Well Water	12
West Hechi	3.9*****		Wells + Hongshu River	22
Bama Yao	4.2		Wells + Pan Yang River	32

* Tiribi Tuff is near population center[146,150]   ** Based upon 6-8 vs. 3-4 glasses of water a day
*** Based upon average river temperatures[142]   ****Centenarian prevalence 6/100K in year 2000
***** Centenarian prevalence 33/100K in year 2000

Okinawa, Japan

Okinawan Centenarian Study - The Japanese Ministry of Health became interested in the extreme longevity of Okinawan's and began the Okinawan Centenarian Study in 1975. It is currently the world's longest continuously running study of centenarians. World-wide interest in the Okinawan longevity region began in 1979 when Shigechiyo Izuma was crowned the world's ultimate survivor in the game of life by the Guinness Book of World Records. At age 115 he was claimed to be the oldest human in the world. He lived in the Kagoshima Prefecture that includes Okinawa and had led a robust and productive life retiring as a farmer at 105 and ultimately lived to 120. His life-story interested people around the world who wanted to emulate him.

Although the Guinness Book of World records continues to regard Mr. Izuma as the oldest man ever documented[89], investigation by Japanese demographers revealed, in all likelihood, Mr. Izuma had "inherited" his first name and with it the prior census data from an older deceased sibling. Mr. Izuma was actually 10 years younger than he claimed[90]. But amazingly he did live to 110. This case of misrepresentation underscores the importance of careful verification in identifying longevity regions.

Okinawan Longevity Region Verification – The longevity regions and their centenarians attract world-wide attention that ultimately brings in tourist dollars. For this reason, there are many "want-to-be" longevity regions but to qualify there must be a published systematic validation of centenarian prevalence. In 2006 The Japanese Ministry of Health scientists performed comprehensive age validation on a subset (8%) of the total Okinawan centenarian population[91]. Careful scrutiny of birth and death records and other age-related documents is necessary to support longevity claims. Demographers confirmed there were four times as many Okinawan centenarians per capita than those on the Japanese mainland. In 2006 Okinawa had 740 centenarians of which 84% were women in a population of 1.3 million[91,92].

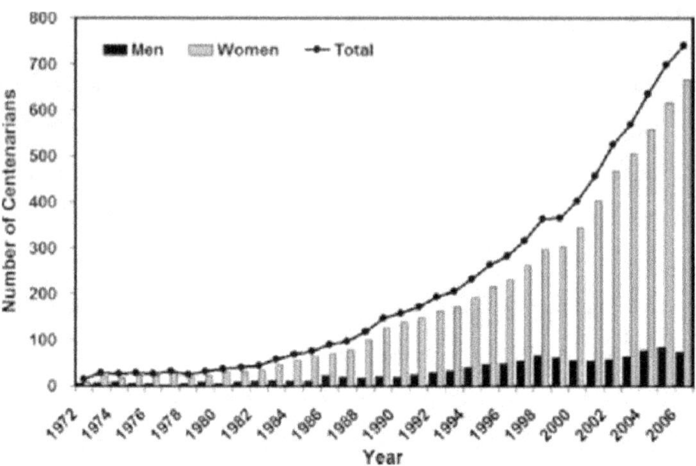

Figure 9. Number of Centenarians in Okinawa from 1972 to 2006[91]

Why Okinawa is a Longevity Region - From 1974 to 2006 the number of centenarians in Okinawa grew 300-fold (see Figure 9) while the population only grew 1.3-fold from 1 million to 1.3 million[93]. In order to discover what was causing this rise in longevity the Ministry of Health gerontologists conducted the largest double-blind study evaluating factors considered at the time to contribute to longevity including: exercise, genetics, diet, caloric restriction, stress reduction, and other lifestyle habits. Results of this study found some unquantifiable but relevant differences between Okinawan's and mainland Japanese:

- Okinawan's in general do have an ikigai or sense of purpose.
- Okinawan centenarians have maintained an average body mass index (BMI) that ranges from 18 to 22, with lean being less than 23. Eating fewer calories has been shown to keep BMI low and increase lifespan[94]. Also drinking OSA rich water lowers BMI[1].
- Okinawan centenarians maintain social bonds with small groups of friends for life.
- Okinawan centenarians have genetic polymorphisms of the human leukocyte antigen (HLA) gene that place them at lower risk for inflammatory and autoimmune diseases[95].

These cultural and genetic differences between Okinawa and mainland Japan had existed well over a century before 1974 and unlikely account for the rapid rise in centenarians after 1974. However, the most important clues to Okinawan longevity are the very low mortality risks from cardiovascular disease (e.g., heart disease and stroke), dementia, and certain cancers on Okinawa. These terminal diseases are major causes of death worldwide and aluminum has been shown to be a causal factor[1].

Heart Disease - Researchers found that Okinawans have low homocysteine as compared to westerners. This low homocysteine may account for why Okinawans have less atherosclerotic narrowing and calcification and an 80% reduced risk for coronary heart disease compared to westerners. An autopsy of a 100-year-old Okinawan women in 2004 revealed normal age-associated changes in her heart but remarkably her coronary vessels were free of atherosclerotic narrowing and calcification[96]. Autopsy reports on non-Okinawan centenarians show coronary vessel narrowing in 66% of centenarians and coronary calcification in 84 to 97% of centenarians[97,98].

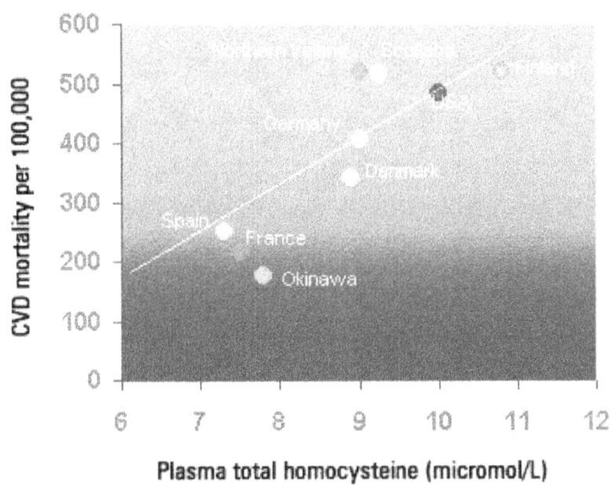

Figure 10 – Cardiovascular disease (CVD) mortality versus plasma homocysteine by country[99]

High levels of plasma homocysteine are correlated with increased risk of cardiovascular disease including stroke and atherosclerosis (a.k.a. hardening of the arteries)[1]. Homocysteine is a causal factor of atherosclerosis[1]. Aluminum ions increase plasma total homocysteine by inhibiting the activation of an enzyme (i.e., methionine synthase) that converts homocysteine to harmless methionine. Insulin-like growth factor normally stimulates methionine synthase. But aluminum ions inhibit this stimulation at levels found *in vivo* (i.e., biphasic: 50% inhibition at 2.7 parts per trillion equivalent to 0.1 nano moles per liter and 50% inhibition at 2.7 parts per billion)[100,101].

Dementia - A prevalence survey showed even in their late 90s Okinawans had lower dementia rates than comparable populations in both the U.S.A. and Japan[102].

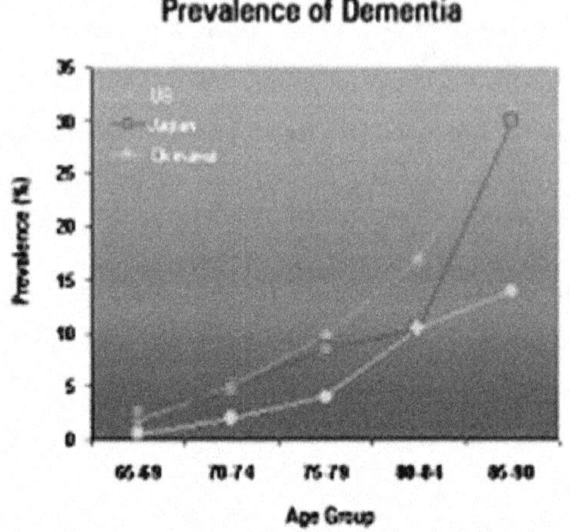

Figure 11 – Showing that the prevalence of dementia is lower on Okinawa[102-104]

The most common types of dementia are vascular dementia (e.g., vascular disease and stroke) and Alzheimer's disease. Aluminum is a causal factor for both of these types of dementia[1].

Cancer – In 1996 Okinawans had 50% less breast and prostate cancer than mainland Japanese and more than 80% less breast and prostate cancer than recorded in the U.S.A. per 100,000 people (see Table 5)[105,106].

Table 5. – Yearly Cancer Deaths per 100,000 People[105-106]		
Location	**Breast Cancer**	**Prostate Cancer**
Okinawa	6	4
Japan	11	8
USA	33	28

The risk of breast and prostate cancer is significantly increased if the *BRCA1* tumor suppression gene's expression is reduced, eliminated, or corrupted by a germ cell mutation[107]. Germ cells when fully developed become sperm or ovum. *BRCA1* expression is reduced or undetectable in the majority of high grade, ductal breast cancers[108]. When expressed, *BRCA1* produces a breast cancer type 1 susceptibility protein called BRCA1. This protein is responsible for error-free repair of double-strand breaks in DNA. When DNA is not repaired properly, there is an increased risk of cancer[109]. Aluminum ions lower the expression of *BRCA1* and thereby increase the risk of breast and prostate cancer[110,111]. OSA in drinking water facilitates the elimination of aluminum in urine and perspiration preventing the development of breast and prostate cancer.

Okinawan Drinking Water - Professor Jun Kobayashi of Okayama University, who had been studying the water of Japan and globally for 40 years, suggested Okinawan longevity might be due to the unique drinking water in Okinawa. Unlike some of the other islands of Japan that formed as a result of volcanos, Okinawa was formed from limestones. These limestones contain high levels of calcium silicate (Ca_2SiO_4) a silicate dissolvable as OSA, not insoluble silica (SiO_2) in quartz and mica as found in plutonic granite from volcanic activity[14]. When it rains on Okinawa, the water filters through the limestone formation being enriched with minerals, such as OSA. The water Okinawans drink, give to their animals, and water their gardens is rich in OSA.

Okinawan drinking water sources and the percentage of drinking water they supply in 2014[16] :

- River water reservoirs 81%
- River water 12%
- Groundwater 6.4%
- Converted seawater 0.7%

Northern Okinawa is mountainous and the location of most of the island's rivers. Therefore, dams and reservoirs are situated in northern regions and this water is supplied to the southern part of the island that has a larger population density. There are three limestones in the Ryukyu Island Archipelago: Naha, Yontan, and Machinato. Naha Limestone has the highest percentage of calcium silicate of the three limestones and coral as shown in Table 6. Okinawa Island rests on a 50-meter-thick layer of Naha Limestone that is exposed up to elevations of approximately 170 meters[15]. Because calcium silicate in limestone is 0.01% soluble in water, the springs, streams, and rivers in contact with this limestone are enriched with OSA[14]. The primary component of all three of these limestones is calcium carbonate (a.k.a. calcite) that is only soluble in weak acids[14]. Therefore, in rain or spring water near neutrality, primarily the calcium silicate dissolves.

Table 6. Calcium Silicate in Ryukyu Limestones and Corals[14]				
	Naha	**Yontan**	**Machinato**	**Coral**
Ca_2SiO_4	21.41%	7.34%	3.35%	0.43%

These percentages are averages of ~50 samples of limestone and 24 samples of coral[14].

The river waters in the northern Kunigami District of Okinawa have low conductivity (less than 150uS/cm) and therefore low carbonate levels[112]. The river waters in the southern Shimajiri District of Okinawa have high conductivity (400 to 900uS/cm) and high carbonate levels[112]. Low conductivity river waters in northern Okinawa are considered "non-carbonate waters" and have much more dissolved silicate than river waters in southern Okinawa as shown in Table 7[14].

Table 7. OSA in Okinawan Drinking Water Sources[14,112]			
Source	**Carbonate**	**Conductivity μS/cm**	**OSA ppm**
Southern Rivers & Reservoirs	High	400-900	7
Northern Rivers & Reservoirs	Low	110-144	40

Since most Okinawans live in the southern part of the island, they drank water with low levels of dissolved silica until a water system was developed to supply northern river and reservoir water to the south. The first Okinawan water system with aqueduct, pumping station, and water treatment began supplying northern water to 3,000 locations in 1933. In 1944 the water supply facility was destroyed in World War II and not reopened until 1951. One of the largest reservoirs in the water supply system is the Fukuji Reservoir located in Northern Kunigami District of Okinawa. This reservoir began supplying drinking water to Okinawans in 1974. The water conductivity of the Fukuji Reservoir varies seasonally from 110 to 144/uS/cm[112]. These water conductivities indicate that this reservoir is filled with low carbonate and high silicate water and has approximately 40ppm per liter of dissolved OSA[14].

Okinawans had the highest survival rates to age 90 of any other longevity region: male 6.6% and female 16.3%[2]. Looking at the history of Okinawa's water system it is likely that these survivors drank 40ppm silica water from 1951 until they eventually died. Professor Kobayashi was right when he postulated that a major factor in Okinawan longevity is in their drinking water. It is very likely that this factor is OSA. OSA facilitates the elimination of aluminum thereby removing from the body a causal factor for cardiovascular disease, vascular dementia, Alzheimer's disease, breast and prostate cancer[1].

Okinawan Hip Fractures – Hip fractures are considered a terminal disease because in the elderly they usually result in permanent immobility and associated health complications. Okinawans have 20% fewer hip fractures than do mainland Japanese and about 40% fewer hip fractures than Americans[113]. The rate of bone mineral density loss was compared between Okinawans and mainland Japanese. It was discovered that for women older than 40 and men older than 50, mainland Japanese lose more calcium from their bones than Okinawans[114]. The higher bone density in older Okinawans is likely due to high levels of OSA in their drinking water. OSA supplementation has been shown to improve bone mineral density by both inhibiting bone mass loss and stimulating bone formation in humans[86-88] and rats[115-117].

Japanese Drinking Water – Is 40ppm of silicate in the drinking water of Okinawa substantially higher than levels of silicate in drinking water on the Japanese mainland? In order to answer this question, we must first define what is mainland Japan. Japan consists of a number of islands the largest of which is called Honshu or "Main Island". Eighty percent of the population of Japan lives on Honshu.

There are two papers that address silica levels in drinking water of Honshu[12,13]. The accuracy and comparability of the data in these two papers was confirmed in two ways. First both papers measured OSA in commercially available Volvic water by either Coradin's yellow or blue procedures[29]. Secondly, I measured OSA in Volvic water using Coradin's blue procedure (see Appendix IV)[1]. All three measurements indicate that Volvic water has 48ppm of OSA within a variation of 3ppm. The Honshu drinking water data is given by prefecture and adjusted for the population of each prefecture in Table 8. There is on average 26ppm of OSA in tap water on the Japanese mainland of Honshu. This is below the 40ppm of OSA in tap water of Okinawa.

Table 8. Silica in Drinking Water of Mainland Japan[12,13]				
Prefecture	SiO₂ ppm	OSA ppm	Population (millions)	Population Adjusted OSA
Fukui	7.6	12.2	0.80	0.27
Gifu	10.6	17	2.07	0.97
Ibaraki	17	27.2	2.96	2.23
Kanagawa	24.7	39.5	9.07	9.91
Kurobe	11.2	17.9	0.04	0.02
Osaka	5.3	8.5	2.69	0.63
Saitama	13.7	21.9	7.15	4.33
Tokyo	17.7	28.3	9.27	7.25
Toyama	7.2	11.5	1.09	0.35
Wakayama	6.8	10.9	1.02	0.31
Totals			36.16	26ppm

Population adjusted OSA equals prefecture population times ppm OSA divided by 36.16 ppm

Okinawa is not the only southern island in Japan with high levels of OSA in their drinking water. The Kagoshima Prefecture in the southwest corner of Kyushu Island also has high levels of OSA in their drinking water. For example, two cities in this Prefecture, Kagoshima City and Kirishima City, have 100ppm and 126ppm of OSA in their drinking water respectively[13]. The average OSA in tap water taken at 12 sites in the Kagoshima Prefecture on Kyushu was 85ppm[13]. The Kagoshima Prefecture deserves study as an undiscovered but potential longevity region. The Kagoshima Prefecture extends south to Okinawa and includes a number of smaller islands in the Ryukyu Island Archipelago. One of these small islands is Kikaijima that is approximately half-way between Okinawa and Kyushu.

Kikaijima Island in the Kagoshima Prefecture is where **Nabi Tajima lived when on September 15th 2017 she became the oldest person on earth!** Nabi was born on August 4th 1900 in the town of Araki in the western most part of Kikaijima Island. She lived her later life in the city of Kikai located on Kikaijima Island. Her age was validated by the Guinness Book of World Records. Nabi became a member of an exclusive group of 46 **supercentenarians** on earth who were over 110 years old in September of 2017. Nabi died on April 21st 2018 at the age of 117.

Conclusion of Okinawa Longevity Region- A longevity region is an area of the world where people have a statistically better chance of living beyond 90 than those living just outside the longevity region. A litmus test for longevity regions is an area where there is a higher density of centenarians in the population. Okinawa passed this litmus test in 1975. The Okinawan Centenarian Study started in 1975 and began looking at why the people of Okinawa have been able to avoid common terminal diseases unlike mainland Japan and the U.S.A. They found that four diseases that increase the risk of mortality were significantly reduced in Okinawa:

- Cardiovascular disease as evidenced by low levels of plasma homocysteine
- Cancer as evidence by low rates of breast and prostate cancer
- Dementia as evidenced by low rates of Alzheimer's disease
- Higher bone density as evidenced by lower incidence of hip fracture

Aluminum is a likely causal factor of all of these diseases (see Chapter 5). Silica water, as OSA in drinking water, has been shown to facilitate aluminum elimination[73]. One of the largest epidemiology studies performed to date has shown that OSA in drinking water lowers the risk of Alzheimer's disease[118]. OSA in drinking water has been shown to improve bone mineral density by both inhibiting bone mass loss and stimulating bone formation in humans[86-88] and rats[115-117].

Table 9 compares the level of OSA in drinking water with health statistics in Okinawa, mainland Japan, and the U.S.A. indicating that higher OSA leads to better health and greater longevity.

Table 9. Correlation Between OSA in Tap Water and Human Health and Longevity							
		Deaths per 100,000			μmol/L	% of 60-79s reaching 90	
Location	ppm OSA tap water	Alzheimer Disease	Breast Cancer	Prostate Cancer	Homo cysteine	Male Survival	Female Survival
Okinawa	40	2.0	6	4	8	6.6	16.3
Japan mainland	26	4.2	11	8	11	3.5	10.5
U.S.A.	11	45.6	33	28	10	2.7	7.7

Date for Table 9 came from Tables 4, 5, and 8, Figures 10 and 11, and reference 460

My chance meeting with Martha R. A. Fields at the local library and this data on Okinawa motivated me to continue my detective work examining the levels of OSA in the drinking water of the other longevity regions. In the next sections of Chapter 3 data on OSA levels of drinking water in the other longevity regions is discussed.

Sardinia and Villagrande, Italy

Sardinia, Italy is a beautiful island in the Mediterranean Sea off the west coast of the Italian mainland. The interior of the island is mountainous and dry. Since the Bronze Age one of the problems with living in this region is the insufficient supply of water. In Sardinia demographers have identified two regions that have a higher density of centenarians than normal in Italy.

- Sardinia longevity region – the entire island
- Villagrande super-longevity region – 14 villages including Villagrande

The Ogliastra is the most mountainous province in Sardinia and the least populous province of Italy with only 57,642 inhabitants. This region is on the Tyrrhenian Sea in eastern Sardinia and hosts some of the most beautiful landscapes in the world. In 2016 the Ogliastra Province was abolished and almost all of its 23 cities joined the Province of Nuoro. There are now 74 villages in the Province of Nuoro. The inner mountainous area of the former Ogliastra Province is the southern part of Barbagia. The people of Barbagia live on the slopes of the Supremonte Mountains and work as sheep herders and farmers.

The village of Villagrande is 50km south southeast of the city of Nuoro. The people of southern Barbagia living in 14 villages, including Villagrande, have extreme longevity when compared to the longevity of Sardinian people. This is impressive because Sardinian males have nearly twice the longevity of Italians living on the mainland in Italy (see Table 4). Possibly even more impressive is the fact that people living in Barbagia are some of the poorest people in Italy.

Sardinian Centenarian Validation - A traditional Sardinian greeting is "A Kent'Annos" or the acronym "AKEA" that means "a hundred years". In 1999 the AKEA I study of Sardinia's centenarians identified 233 potentially eligible centenarians who were born from 1880 to 1900[119]. In order to validate these centenarians a multidimensional home interview was conducted of 141 of the 233 potentially eligible centenarians and their locations in 1999 are indicated with black and gray solid-colored dots on map on the left of Figure 12. The locations of those not interviewed are indicated with black and gray circles on the map on the left of Figure 12. From this data it is apparent that most of the centenarians live in the central mountainous region of Sardinia.

Villagrande Centenarian Validation – The data from the AKEA I study was used to identify an area in the Province of Nuoro for the AKEA II Nuoro centenarian validation study. This area has the highest probability of any one born to reach 100 years of age (called the Extreme Longevity Index or ELI)[120]. This super-longevity region is in the vicinity and to the northeast of Villagrande, including 13 other villages in Southern Barbagia and the former Ogliastra Province. These villages are in the most mountainous area in Sardinia. The total population of the area at the time of the study was approximately 40,000. The inhabitants were engaged in pastoral and agricultural activities and followed a relatively traditional life style. During 1880 to 1900, 17,965 people were born in the Villagrande super-longevity region and 91 of these people (47 men and 44 women) would reach the age of 100. The age of each centenarian was validated according to accepted rules and criteria[2,120]. The approximate 1 to 1 ratio of female to male centenarians in this super-longevity region is unique as the ratio is usually closer to 5 to 1 as it is in Okinawa[121].

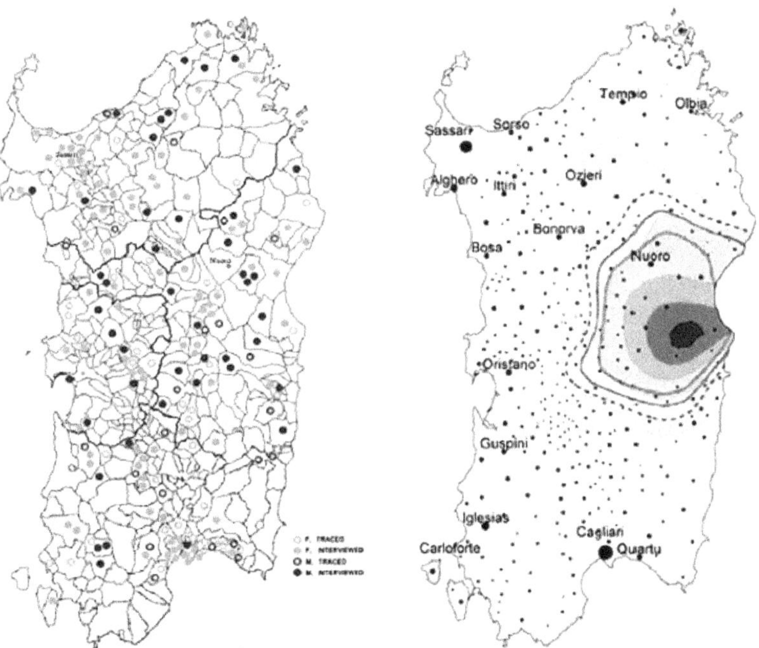

Figure 12. Left is Centenarian Place of Residence in Sardinia[120] and on Right is Map of ELI. The darkened area is the Super-Longevity Region of Villigrande[2,120]

Sardinian Drinking Water – Currently ninety percent of the drinking water in Sardinia comes from approximately 40 artificial lakes made by damming the rivers of the island. Data collected over many decades have shown most of these lakes are eutrophic and dominated by cyanobacteria[122]. In the mountains of Sardinia these artificial lakes were filled with a mixture of water from springs and limited surface water runoff. There are two types of springs in this area:

- Karst Springs
- Thermal Springs

Karst springs are fed from relatively shallow aquifers and underground streams mixed with some surface water runoff[123]. Karst springs usually supply drinking water with less than 10ppm of OSA and can be contaminated with animal and human waste[124].

An example of karst springs is the Su Gologone springs, Sa Vena and Sa Vena Manna. They are in the Gulf of Orosi karst area covering more than 210 square miles[123]. These springs are fed from the Supramonte Aquifer that is located under the Guthiddai Valley at the northeastern foot of Mount Udde (806m)[124]. Water from the Sa Vena spring supplies drinking water to approximately16,000 inhabitants of the villages of Oliena and Dorgali[124]. The waters from these springs were tested from December 2010 to June of 2011 and found to contain on average 6.5ppm of OSA[124]. The flow rate of this spring is seasonally variable from 120 liters/sec during low flow to 5,000 liters/sec during normal floods[125].

Thermal Springs are fed from deep geothermal waters that well up to the surface in the area of geological faults. Before the construction of dams creating artificial lakes, thermal springs were desirable for drinking water as they were less susceptible to both seasonal flow variation and surface runoff contamination than karst springs. OSA in thermal springs in Sardinia is on average 41 to 62ppm as shown in Table 10. Thermal springs in Sardinia vary in water temperature from 15 to 58°C (60 to 136°F)[10]. The lower levels of OSA in some rivers of Sardinia are due to karst springs and surface runoff from rain diluting the OSA from thermal springs that flow into rivers.

Table 10. Dissolved Silica in Thermal Springs and Rivers of Sardinia[9,10]			
Springs & Rivers	**Location**	**Date of Sampling**	**OSA ppm**
3 Springs	Logudoro Fault	Feb. 1997	25-68 (52 avg.)
3 Springs	E. Carpidono Fault	Feb. 1997	21-69 (53 avg.)
3 Springs	Central Graben	Feb. 1997	33-48 (41 avg.)
4 Springs	W. Carpidono Fault	Feb. 1997	23-61 (45 avg.)
3 Springs	Capoterra Fault	Feb. 1997	54-69 (62 avg.)
Padrongianu River	N.E. Sardinia	June 2008	26-31 (29 avg.)
Mascari River	N. Sardinia	Feb. & July 2009	15-24 (20 avg.)
Tributary of Mascari	N. Sardinia	Feb. & July 2009	8-12 (11 avg.)
Pauli Gippe River	W. Sardinia	August 2008	20
Tanui River	W. Sardinia	August 2008	27
Iscas River	W. Sardinia	August 2008	26

There are two sources of OSA in the thermal springs of Sardinia: Late Mesozoic\Eosene limestone in East-Central Sardinia and alluvial deposits in the area of the Campidano and Capoterra faults in Southwestern Sardinia[34]. In East-Central Sardinia the most likely source of OSA is diatom fossils in the upper layers of the Late Mesozoic\Eosene limestone plate (shaded as brick-work on the map in the left of Figure 13). After the extinction of dinosaurs 66 million years ago diatoms diversified and multiplied in the world's oceans becoming the dominate-sink for OSA in the oceans at the expense of other organisms that require OSA, including both the radiolarian and reef-building sponge population[126,127]. Therefore, this limestone, like Naha Limestone in Okinawa, is high in silicate and low in aluminum as described in the next section of this chapter on Villagrande drinking water.

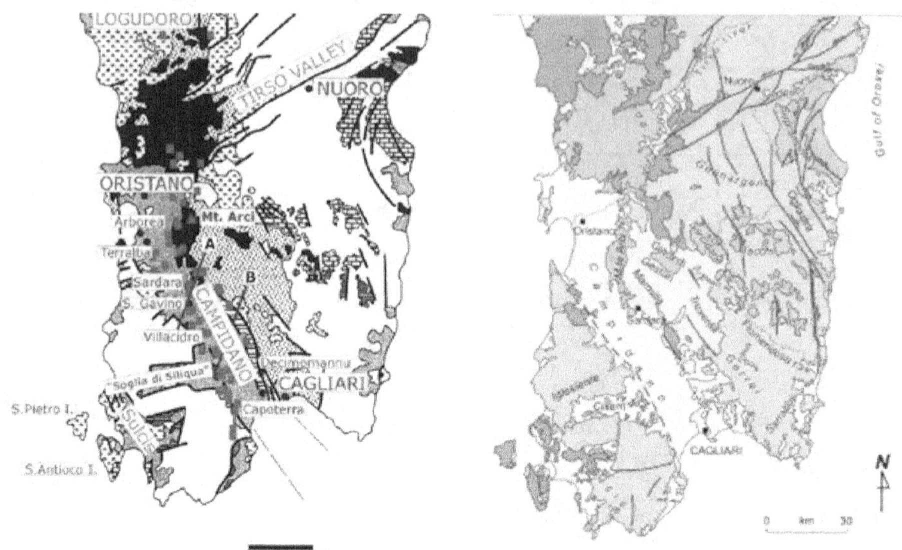

Figure 13. Southern Sardinia Geological Features: **Map on Left** - black lines are geological faults, white zones are Paleozoic crystalline basement, brick-work shaded areas are Mesozoic\Eocene limestone plate, and red squares are selected thermal springs[9]. **Map on Right** - Red lines are more geological faults. Blue shaded areas south and east of Nuoro are Mesozoic\Eocene limestone plates. Villagrande is 50km south southeast of Nuoro at the intersection of a fault and silicate rich fossilized diatomic late Mesozoic\Eocene limestone[34].

Villagrande Drinking Water – Like the Naha limestone in Northern Okinawa, the late Mesozoic\Eocene limestone plate underlies the Villagrande super-longevity region providing this area with OSA rich drinking water (see Figure 13 and Table 10). Although there are numerous OSA rich thermal springs in Sardinia, this late Mesozoic\Eocene limestone adjacent to faults is unique to the super-longevity region. The two maps in Figure 13 show many geological faults and thermal springs in southern Sardinia. In an area overlapping with the super-longevity region there are many geochemically active faults running through or adjacent to late Mesozoic\Eocene limestone plates including the Tirso River fault north of Nuoro. Villagrande is 50km south southeast of Nuoro at the intersection of a fault and silica rich fossilized diatomic late Mesozoic\Eocene limestone (see Figure 13)[34].

Some thermal springs and rivers near Tirso Fault and the City of Nuoro were analyzed for OSA from 1997-2010[9-11]. Results of this analysis are in Table 11. Of the 23 thermal springs analyzed all but three had OSA greater than 48ppm[11]. In one of the springs with low OSA the aluminum level was 650ppb but in the rest of the springs, aluminum ranged from 6 to 40ppb with an average of 15ppb[11]. From this data it is likely that those people who were born during the period 1880 to 1900 in the mountains of East-Central Sardinia, including Villagrande, were exposed to high levels of OSA and low levels of aluminum from their conception to middle age assuming they drank water from thermal springs.

Table 11. Dissolved Silica in Thermal Springs and Rivers of Super-Longevity Region[9-11]			
Springs & Rivers	**Location**	**Date of Sampling**	**OSA ppm**
18 Springs	20km from Nuoro	May 2001	44 – 64 (51 avg.)
3 Springs	20km from Nuoro	May 2001	24–37 (32 avg.)
1 Spring	Tirso River Fault	1985-2001	59 – 67 (64 avg.)
1 Spring	Tirso River Fault	August 1997	59
Tirso River	22km from Nuoro	May 2001	10
		April 2009	25 – 27 (26 avg.)
Mannu River	17km from Nuoro	May 2001	11
		August 2008	37

The two rivers tested, Tirso and Mannu, both had medium levels of aluminum, 69 and 41ppb respectively[11]. The level of total dissolved solids (TDS) in the rivers and springs is considered low[8]. The TDS in rivers was approximately half that of the thermal springs (i.e., 250ppm versus 500ppm)[11]. This indicates the water from thermal springs that flows into the rivers is probably diluted with water from karst springs and surface runoff.

Villagrande Drinking Water History - The extreme longevity index (ELI) of the Villagrande super-longevity region indicates that newborns born from 1880 to 1900 in this region were twice as likely to reach 100 as being born anywhere else in Sardinia during that time period[120]. In

1880 to 1950 the artificial lakes were not yet built and water in the Southern Barbagia region was primarily supplied from local thermal springs. For instance, the dam creating Lago Bau Muggens near Villagrande was not built until 1949.

Because of the dryness of the region around Villagrade it is likely that the 14 villages in this super-longevity region were built close to sources of pure drinking water uncontaminated with surface water runoff, such as thermal springs. From the data in Table 11 it is likely that these thermal springs contained very high levels of OSA (i.e., 44 to 64ppm) and low levels of aluminum (i.e., averaging 15ppb) .

Nuragic Wells

The Nuragic civilization lived in the mountains of Sardinia from Aegean Bronze Age (18th century BC) to the 2nd century AD. These people were dedicated to the "cult of water" and built holy wells to both protect and access the spring-fed water supplies in these regions. Examples are the Su Tempiesu and the Noddule holy wells in the Province of Nuoro. The architecture of these Nuragic holy wells consists of a circular room with a small hole in the summit and monumental staircase connecting the entrance to a subterranean room.

The main role of these structures was to allow for the protection and collection of water from thermal springs.

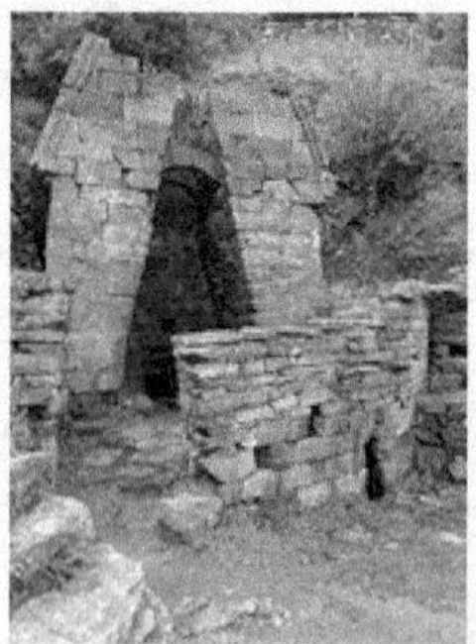 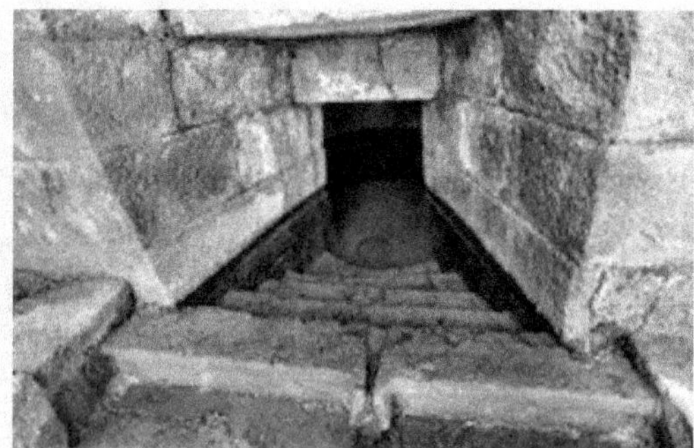

Figure 14. The Su Tempiesu Nuragic Well outside the Village of Orune near Nuoro, Sardinia

Italian Drinking Water – I frequently visited Italy in the early 1970's on business and was amazed at the amount of bottled water being consumed as it was almost unheard of in the U.S.A. at that time. In addition, there was a complete list of all minerals in the water, including silica, on the bottle's label. I remember that the information on the label was an important part of meal-time conversation. The trend in Italian bottled water usage has risen approximately 10-fold from 1970 to 2000[8], as shown in Figure 15. This is the same time period over which survival-to-90 rates were measured in the longevity regions and their parent countries as indicated in Table 3.

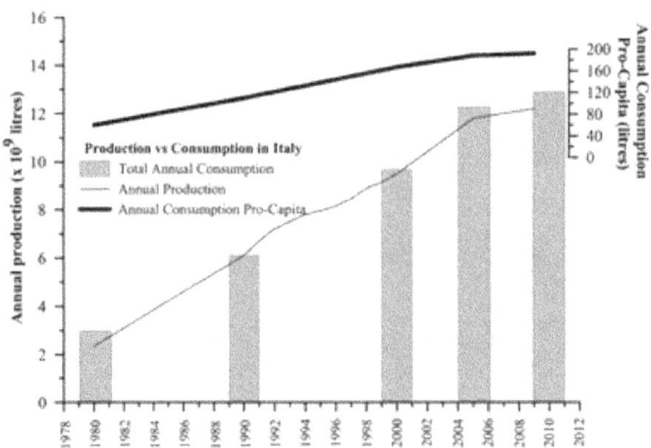

Figure 15. Annual production and consumption per-capita of bottled mineral water in Italy[8]

Over 400 brands of water bottled and sold currently in Italy were tested for OSA content. The median concentration was 17ppm with half the brands less than 17ppm and half the brands higher than 17ppm of OSA[8]. The total range of OSA was 1 to 220ppm OSA. There are no published OSA levels for tap water in Italy. However, since these 400 brands of mineral water are basically the same as regional tap water, this bottled water likely contains the same levels of OSA as tap waters in Italy.

Conclusion of Sardinian and Villagrandian Longevity Regions - The drinking water in both the Sardinia longevity region and Villagrande super-longevity region contains significantly higher levels of OSA than do average mainland Italian bottled and non-bottled drinking waters. The Villagrande super-longevity region is unique because it geographically coincides[2] with an underlying layer of silica rich fossilized diatomic late Mesozoic\Eocene limestone that is intersected with numerous faults (see Figures 12 and 13)[9,34]. This makes it likely that from 1880 to 1949 the Villagrande drinking water was high in OSA (51ppm avg.) and low in aluminum (15ppb avg.). During this period of time the future centenarians who were born between 1980 and 2000 had been conceived and grew into adulthood.

The mobility of the people of Villagrande is very low. Of the 1,957 people born in Villagrande from 1876 to 1912 only 10% died outside of Villagrande[121]. This translates into a lifetime spent drinking water high in OSA and low in aluminum for 90% of the residents of Villagrande. This was true at least until the reservoir called Lago Bau Muggens was constructed in 1949. This sets the people of Villagrande apart from Okinawans born during the same period who did not have high OSA water until 1933 with an interruption from 1944 to 1951. This means Okinawans did not have high OSA water until middle age. Could this account for why there is a 5 to 1 female to male ratio of centenarians in Okinawan versus a 1 to1 ratio of centenarians in Villagrande?

Autism may provide a clue to answer this question. The female to male ratio of children with autism has been generally found to be 1 to 4 indicting boys are more likely than girls to have autism[128]. Approximately 50% of the children with autism, mostly boys, have increased intestinal permeability that is not seen in children without autism[129]. Aluminum has been found at much higher levels than normal in the hair and brains of children with autism[130-132]. From these observations aluminum may be a causal factor of autism and boys likely absorb in general more aluminum than girls[1].

If boys absorb more aluminum than girls, then drinking water with high levels of OSA may benefit boys more than girls. Since chronic aluminum toxicity has been linked to heart disease, the advantage for boys in drinking OSA rich water may extend to a greater decrease in male versus female heart disease in midlife. Therefore, OSA in drinking water could benefit the longevity of boys more than girls and could account for Villagrande's unique 1 to 1 female to male ratio of centenarians not seen in the Okinawan longevity region.

Ikaria, Greece

Ikaria is a small mountainous island in the Aegean Sea that is traversed by the Aetheras Mountain range with a peak elevation of 1,037 meters (3,400 feet). It is believed to be named after Icarus who flew too close to the sun and melted his wax wings falling into the ocean near Ikaria. Although Icarus is not an icon of longevity, the approximately 8,300 residents of Ikaria are almost free of dementia and some chronic diseases and on average live longer than people on the mainland of Greece. A number of health springs on Ikaria were first observed and described as having curative powers by Herodotous (484-425 BC)[133]. The current residents of Ikaria primarily live in the plains near the coast where these thermal springs are located.

Ikaria Centenarian Validation – In Ikaria census data and age-at-death statistics were obtained from Greece. For the very old no birth records could be found. Therefore, age validation could only be done by exhaustive interviews with all those 90 and above[134]. This was primarily performed on the north side of the island. The percentage of people over age 90 living on Ikaria was much higher than the percentage of people over 90 in the mainland Italian population[133]. The average age at death from natural causes on Ikaria is nearly 10 years greater than in Greece[135]. In addition, Ikarians have approximately 20% lower rates of cancer, 50% lower rates of heart disease, 25% less dementia, and less depression[137].

Ikaria Epidemiology Study - From June to October of 2009 the Ikaria Epidemiology Study took place in Ikaria. This study was organized by Christina Chrysohoou and Demosthenes B. Panagiotakos of the Harokopio University and C. I. Stefanadis of the Department of Cardiology of Athens Medical School. This was the first academic study of dietary and lifestyle factors on Ikaria that might account for the islander's longevity. The study involved first surveying 1,470 Ikarians and testing 343 men and 330 women all over age 65 with 79 of them over age 90. Everyone in the study was a permanent resident of the island. In addition to socio-demographic, lifestyle, physical activity, and dietary characteristics, cardiovascular risk factors were evaluated including: hypertension, diabetes, hypercholesterolemia, and obesity, and biochemical parameters relating to cardiovascular risk[133,135].

Ikarian Sociodemographic and Lifestyle Statistics – As part of the Ikaria Epidemiology Study a group of Ikarians over the age of 80 were interviewed with respect to their behaviors and lifestyles (89 males and 98 females)[133]. The study revealed the following four modifiable lifestyle factors were linked to the "secrets" of longevity on Ikaria:

- **Smoking Cessation** – Only 17% of men and 7% of women currently smoked while 82% of men and 25% of women were former smokers
- **Daily Moderate Physical Activity** - 89% of men and 70% of women performed moderate to high daily physical activity and only 0.8% of men and 0.3% of women owned a car
- **Avoiding Lack of Sleep** – Mid-day naps supplemented a good night's sleep
- **Moderate Alcohol Consumption** – Daily wine consumption was on average 6oz. for men and 4oz. for women.

These causes of human longevity are all recommended for good physical and mental health[1]. But are they sufficiently unique to set Ikaria apart from Greece? Based upon the data presented so far in this book there is an additional lifestyle factor that must be considered important for longevity:

- **Drinking OSA Rich Water**

Ikaria Drinking Water – In the memories of some elderly Ikarians living in the villages of Agios Kirikos (population 3,500) there was "Immortal Water" sold by a wandering water seller with his donkey loaded with water pitchers. This "Immortal Water" came from a famous local spring called "Athanatou Nero" that was hidden amidst large granite rocks. The water is still very tasty and is rumored to have therapeutic values. There are springs like this throughout Ikaria and as it turns out they may be an important factor accounting for Ikarian longevity.

Along the southeastern coast of Ikaria there are two types of thermal springs: cool water thermal springs and hot water thermal springs (see Table 10). In the region of the villages of Agios Kirikos, Chrisostomos, Plagia, and Petropoulan six cool water thermal springs were tested for OSA and their waters were found to contain on average 35ppm with a range of 18 to 58ppm[7]. In the region north of Agios Kirikos nine hot water thermal springs were tested and found to contain too much chloride to be potable. In spite of this they did contain on average 34ppm of OSA with a range of 22 to 51ppm[7]. The source of the chloride in the hot thermal springs is likely due to sea water intrusion[7]. The cool springs contain mineral water diluted with rainwater and the hot springs contain mineral water diluted with seawater[7]. This data is summarized in Table 12 and the locations of the thermal springs are indicted on the map in Figure 16.

Table 12. OSA in Cool and Hot Thermal Springs of Ikaria[7]				
Springs	Temperature °C	OSA ppm	Chloride ppm	Conductivity µS/cm
Cool #8-11 and 14-15	18.6 avg. (17-21)	35 (18-58)	40 (29-47)	308 (212-438)
Hot #1-7 and 12-13	37 avg. (21-58)	34 (22-51)	15,880 (0.8-22K)	37,630 (3-50K)

The springs of Ikaria have the same amount of OSA independent of their widely different chloride level and conductivities. This is likely due to the springs of Ikaria arising from similar geology as shown in Figure 16. Ikaria is known for its numerous thermal springs that are classified as some of the most radioactive springs in the world[7]. The radioactivity is due to radium in the water acquired from radioactive minerals in the rocks that come in contact with the water.

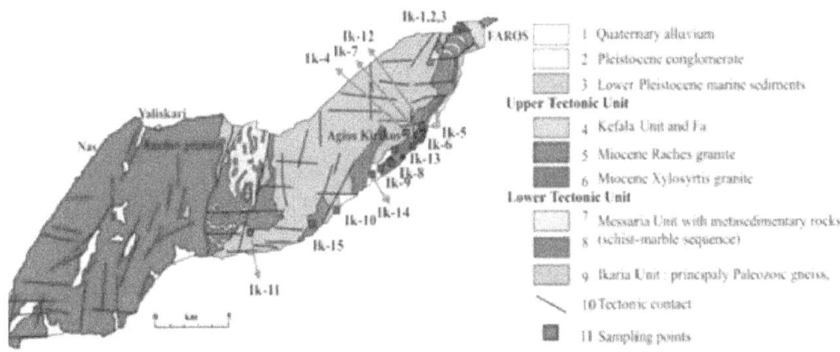

Figure 16. Geological map of Ikaria and location of faults and cool and hot springs[7]

Ikarian Geology – The bulk of the population of Ikaria live in the northeast half of the island. Underlying this portion of the island are two geological formations: Ikaria Unit, principally Paleozoic gneiss, and Messaria Unit, principally interleaved schist and marble. The Paleozoic gneiss has a layered structure and could be of either igneous or sedimentary origin. If this gneiss is of sedimentary origin, then it might be rich in silica and made of radiolarian fossils that evolved and dominated the world's oceans in the Paleozoic Era. The Messaria marble probably contains very little silica. However, Messaria schist is likely finely interleaved with quartz and/or feldspar both of which are rich in silica.

Grecian Drinking Water – In Greece 87% of the potential fresh water is from surface water, such as rivers and reservoirs, and 13% is from ground water, such as wells and springs[137,138]. Water usage in Greece is divided as follows[138,139]:

- 86% - Agriculture – Irrigation
- 10% - Domestic – Drinking Water
- 4% - Industrial

The drinking water of Greece has been methodically tested for nutrients and environmental contaminates but not for silica[138-140]. Also, some of the rivers of Greece have been tested for nitrate and phosphate but not for silica[141]. This has left researchers to derive silica levels indirectly from environmental factors such as river water temperature. Rivers of the world and those that drain into the Mediterranean with the usual temperature of 12-20°C have on average 13ppm of OSA within a range of 6 to 20ppm[142].

In order to guarantee drinking water delivery from wet season to dry season, river water flowing into the Mediterranean has been increasingly dammed and stored in reservoirs behind the dams. Since 1965 dams have been built in Greece that have increased the volume of fresh water retention by more than 10 square kilometers (see Figure 17)[142,143]. The longer water is retained in a reservoir the more silica is lost to complexation with sediments or polymerization by cyanobacteria catalyzed by ferrihydrite[20,142]. The net effect is more water retention means less OSA in drinking water taken from reservoirs and rivers downstream from reservoirs.

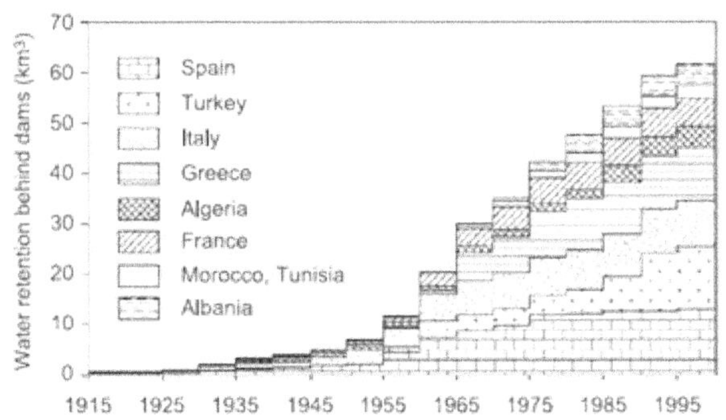

Figure 17. Evolution of water retention behind dams[142,143]

There is an area in Eastern Central Greece called Northern Evia that does have nine wells with potable high OSA water (64 to 100ppm) that is used as drinking water by local villages[144]. These villages have populations too small for any major impact on average Greek health but they might be another undiscovered longevity region. This high OSA water comes from cool (10.6 to 21.5°C) gravity springs not considered to be thermal springs[144]. The source of the silica may be rock layers of uplifted seafloor (ophiolites) that contain mudstones rich in radiolarian fossils[145].

Conclusion of Ikaria Longevity Region - In general the drinking water of Ikaria is more silica rich than are the drinking waters of Greece. By inference this gives Ikarians an advantage as their aluminum excretion by urination and perspiration is facilitated by OSA. Additional advantages are:

- Smoking cessation – tobacco contains aluminum and smoking adds aluminum to the brain
- Moderate physical activity – by not owning cars, Ikarians exercise and perspire resulting in OSA facilitating the excretion of aluminum in perspiration

These advantages are causal factors for approximately 20% lower rates of cancer, 50% lower rates of heart disease, 25% less dementia in Ikaria[135]. Because rates of these diseases are lower, Ikarians live 10 years longer than people living in Greece[135].

Nicoya Peninsula, Costa Rica

In Northwestern Costa Rica the city of Liberia on the Pan-American Highway is the gateway to a beautiful peninsula that is bordered by the Pacific Ocean on the west and the Gulf of Nicoya on the east. The Nicoya Peninsula is currently known as a destination for fine beaches and fantastic surfing.

Henri Pittier, a Swiss geographer and botanist, moved to Costa Rica in 1887. Pittier was a skilled observer of both plants and humans. After visiting the Nicoya Peninsula, he observed that "in no other place are people blessed with such long lives"[146]. Recently Nicoya's longevity has been examined in a population-based sample of elderly Costa Ricans[147]. Pittier's observation was confirmed as Nicoya has a significantly lower death rate ratio compared to the rest of Costa Rica (see Table 4). Since Pittier's observation was made over a century ago, Nicoya's longevity was prevalent even at the time when present day centenarians were born.

This is the first longevity region discussed that is not an island. However, being a peninsula, it is somewhat geographically isolated. The Nicoya longevity region is within the Province of Guanacaste and has a population of 161,000 according to the 2011 census[146]. Most of the Nicoya population is located inland between 100 to 500 meters above sea level and 95% of the population is in three cantons living primarily in the canton's capital city:

Table 13. Cantons of the Nicoya Longevity Region		
Canton	**Capital City**	**Population of Canton**
Carillo	Filadelfia	39,700
Santa Cruz	Santa Cruz	60,500
Nicoya	Nicoya	52,600

The cantons listed in Table 13 are in what is locally called the Guanacaste lowlands. The Tempisque River basin is primarily in the Carillo canton near Filadelfia. Currently the Tempisque River and underground aquifers in the Guanacaste lowlands are insufficient to supply the needed surface and ground water to these cantons. A construction project is beginning in 2018 with the goal of diverting water for human consumption and irrigation from the Piedras

River Reservoir[148]. The first phase of this project is scheduled for completion in 2023. In general this area is mixed forest and agriculture with ground and surface water used for drinking water and crop irrigation.

Nicoya Centenarian Validation – The age validation of the oldest of the old and the assessment of population longevity were based on public voting lists and the birth registry. This registry includes birth dates, naturalizations, and deaths of all Costa Ricans who contacted the civil registration system since its computerization in 1970[149]. Each person was given a unique number at birth or at naturalization that appears on their identification card. The age of the oldest of the old was confirmed with self-reported information at an interview. Data quality and the higher level of longevity on Nicoya compared with the rest of Costa Rico has been confirmed and published[146].

Nicoya Study Results - Nicoyan males have a much greater survival rate to age 90 than do Costa Rican males (see Table 4). This Nicoyan advantage does not extend fully to Nicoyan females who have only a slightly greater survival rate to age 90 than do Costa Rican females (see Table 4). Looking at survival to age 100, a 60-year-old Nicoyan male has a 7 times higher probability of becoming a centenarian than does a 60-year-old Japanese male. The Nicoyan male has a 2.2-year greater life expectancy than does the Japanese male.

The Nicoyan advantage is a death rate ratio of 0.82 versus Costa Rica's 1.0 and is lower (i.e., 0.77) for those that were born and remained in Nicoya (see Table 14)[146]. The Nicoyan advantage does not occur in females, is independent of socio-economic conditions, disappears in out-migrants (those born in Nicoya and at the time of the study living elsewhere), and comes primarily from lower male cardiovascular mortality[146]. Males are also leaner, taller, and suffer fewer disabilities[146]. The higher mortality in out-migrants points to an environmental factor rather than a genetic factor being the cause of the Nicoyan advantage.

Table 14. Migrants Impact on Death Rate Ratio (DDR) [146]

Nicoyan	DDR
Born and Remained in Nicoya	0.77
Migrated into Nicoya	0.93
Migrated out of Nicoya	1.06

Biomarkers of Longevity in Elderly Nicoyans – Biomarkers for about 600 elderly Nicoyans and 4,500 elderly Costa Ricans were analyzed to better understand the Nicoyan advantage[146,147]. The biomarkers found to be significantly different, where Nicoyans are either negatively (i.e., lower) or positively (i.e., higher) than Costa Ricans, are listed in Table 15. Where not indicated the biomarkers were seen in both males and females. Unlike in Okinawa, plasma level of homocysteine was not tested as part of this biomarker survey.

Table 15. Biomarkers for Nicoyan Advantage	
Significant Negative Biomarkers	**Significant Positive Biomarkers**
Activities of Daily Living Disability (ALD)*	Depression (Females Only)
Triglycerides (Males Only)*	Knee Height*
Cognitive Decay*	DHEAS Plasma Level**
Fasting Glucose Plasma Level (Males Only)*	Telomere Length*
Glycated Hemoglobin (Males Only)*	
Total HDL Cholesterol Ratio	
Waist Circumference*	
Body Mass Index (BMI) at ages 80+*	

* These are likely due to OSA lowering aluminum ** DHEAS protects cognition

Aluminum is a likely causal factor of Alzheimer's disease that results in daily living disability (a.k.a. ALD)[1]. OSA also lowers the risk of Alzheimer's disease and prevents ADL disability[1]. Aluminum inhibits the utilization of both glucose and stored fat for energy[1]. This results in higher levels of triglycerides and glycated hemoglobin as well as greater body mass index (a.k.a. BMI) and waist circumference. Both high aluminum levels and triglycerides are causal factors of cardiovascular disease[1]. Drinking silica water (i.e., OSA) facilitates the excretion of aluminum resulting in lower levels of fasting glucose, glycated hemoglobin, and triglycerides in the blood and less BMI, waist circumference, and cardiovascular disease[1]. Information on how aluminum impacts telomere length is described in "Telomere Length as a Biomarker for Longevity" (see Chapter 5).

Nicoya Drinking Water – The Nicoya peninsula is unique as it sets atop the largest area of ophiolites in Costa Rica as shown in Figure 18[150]. Ophiolites are rocks from ancient uplifted sea floor sediment laid down approximately 200 to 40 million years ago. The ophiolite named the Nicoya Complex underling the entire peninsula is formed exclusively of silica-rich intraplate igneous rocks associated with radiolarities[151]. Within the Nicoya Complex is a 50-meter-thick layer called the Punta Conchal Formation. This layer consists of rhythmically thin-stratified radiolarian cherts[152]. Under the central and southern parts of the Nicoya Peninsula there are numerous silica-saturated volcanic tufts and debris with preserved radiolarian fossils[153]. The Nicoya Complex is capped with sandstone that also contains radiolarian skeletons fossilized in radiolarian cherts[151]. It is not surprising with this geology that the surface waters, such as the Tempisque River, and ground waters of Nicoya have high levels of OSA.

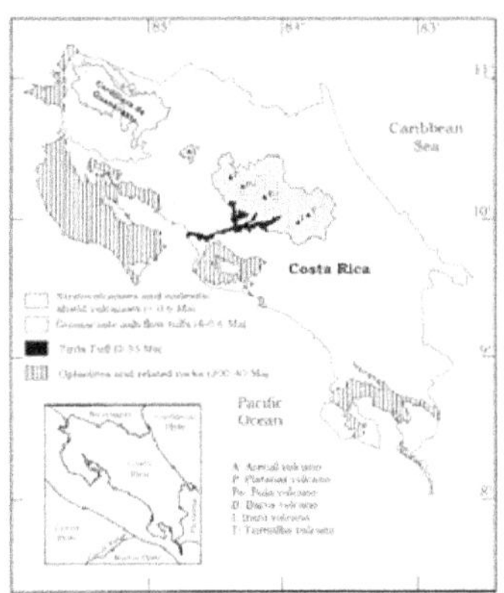

Figure 18. Geological map with the largest area of ophiolites under the Nicoyan Peninsula[150]

The water quality of the Tempisque River has been periodically monitored in both dry and rainy seasons at Guinea in 1980 to 1981 and at Guardia from 1987 to 1991. OSA was one of the factors analyzed and the results are in Table 16[6].

Table 16. OSA in the Tempisque River[6]			
Survey Station	**Season**	**Date**	**OSA ppm**
Guinea	Dry	4/17/1980	112
	Rainy	9/9/1980	94
Guardia	Dry	1/24/1987	124
	Dry	4/25/1987	141
	Dry	2/12/1991	128
	Rainy	8/25/1988	59

The high levels of OSA in the Tempisque River even in the rainy season are similar to levels seen in ground waters of Sardinia and Ikaria.

Costa Rican Drinking Water - Costa Rica is a country with outstanding male and female longevity. Male survivability in Costa Rica is second only to the Villagrande super-longevity region and female survivability in Costa Rica is second only to the Okinawa longevity region (see Table 4). The age-adjusted rate of mortality from cardiovascular disease (CVD), at ages 85 and older, is 20% lower in Costa Rica than the United States[149]. Like Okinawa and Ikaria, Costa Rica also has a low rate of CVD. OSA in drinking water is a likely causal factor in Costa Rica's country-wide longevity.

There are two sources of silica rich substrata in Costa Rica: ophiolites and silicic volcanic ash-flow sheets, such as Tiribi Tuff and the Guanacaste ash-flow tuffs. The areas of these types of deposits are shown in Figure 18[150]. The Tiribi Tuff underlies most of the Valle Central of Costa Rica, currently the most densely populated area in the country with approximately 2.4 million inhabitants (see Figure 19). The Tiribi Tuff contains 59 to 65% silicon dioxide (SiO_2) by weight[150]. Water samples from two streams, the Tizate and Quebrada La Pita, in the area of the Tiribi Tuff were sampled and analyzed at 10 locations in 1998 and found to contain 27.5 to 45.4 ppm of OSA[154]. Drinking water that flows through these deposits is enriched in OSA and the population exposed to this drinking water will accrue health and longevity benefits.

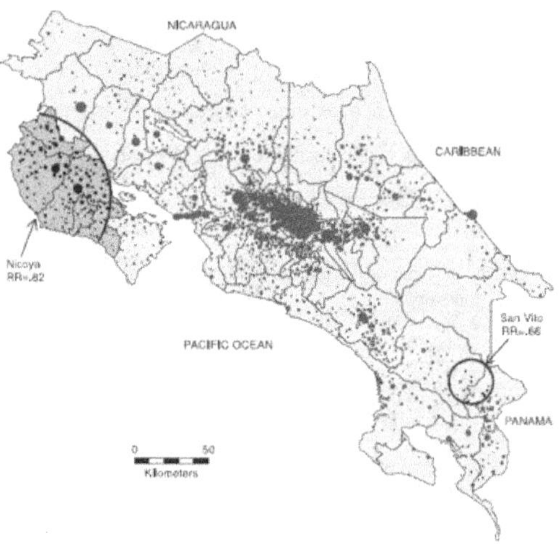

Figure 19. Map of Costa Rica where point size is proportional to population. Canton boarders and Longevity Regions of Nicoya and San Vito are indicated[146].

The city of San Vito and its northern neighboring area circled in Figure 19, like Nicoya, has a population living near silica rich ophiolite deposits. The San Vito area has a population of only 12,000 and in the period from 1990 to 2011 those 70 and older had a very low mortality rate of 0.66 versus 0.82 for Nicoya and 1.0 for Costa Rica[146]. San Vito is at the south end of the Coto Brus Valley at an altitude of 996 meters (3,268 feet) on a high plateau with irregular topography. The Java River flows through the outskirts of San Vito and has been the source of drinking water for the city for many years[155]. The city is located near ophiolite deposits in Southern Costa Rica (see Figure 18) that likely enrich the Java River with OSA.

Conclusion of Nicoya and San Vito Longevity Regions -The Nicoya Peninsula and the area around San Vito are longevity regions in Costa Rica. Both of these longevity regions sit atop or near silica rich ophiolite deposits with the potential of enriching surface and ground water with OSA. It is incredible that there are longevity regions in Costa Rica considering the extreme longevity of Costa Ricans who are also exposed to OSA in their drinking water due to volcanic ash-flow under the Valle Central, where the bulk of the population of Costa Rica resides. The only difference between Costa Rica and its longevity regions may be the level of OSA in the drinking water. Limited water analysis data indicates higher levels of OSA in Nicoyan surface water than in Costa Rican surface water.

The increased longevity in Costa Rica and its longevity regions is primarily due to a low level of male cardiovascular disease (CVD). We have already seen that OSA may be responsible for low CVD in Okinawa and Ikaria. Like Villagrande, being born and remaining in Nicoya is linked to male longevity. People who migrate out of Nicoya have higher mortality than those that remain in Nicoya suggesting that the Nicoyan advantage is environmental and not genetic.

Loma Linda, California, USA

In the 1860's the Seventh-day Adventist church was founded in a sunny pocket of California now called Loma Linda or "beautiful hill" in Spanish. Under the dominant influence of a cofounder, Ellen G. White (1827-1915), the denomination became focused on both missionary and medical work. Church members continue to view health as central to their faith and this view is believed to be why they live longer than non-church members. Between 2000 and 2010 Loma Linda's population grew by 25% to 23,260. Currently Loma Linda is a community of approximately 9,000 Adventists representing about 40% of Loma Linda's population[156]. The community of approximately 35,000 Adventists in California, including those in Loma Linda, is a longevity region when its longevity is viewed in comparison with the Californian population[157].

Loma Linda Centenarian Validation – The U.S.A. census data is not necessarily a reliable source of information. Past U.S.A. censuses have exaggerated the number of American centenarians. The 1980 census, for example, listed approximately double what demographers believe to be the actual prevalence rates of centenarians due to errors, such as either elderly people misreporting their age or 4-year-olds reported as 104 because their birth years were marked wrongly[158,159]. Therefore, in populations that claim more centenarians than normal for the area, careful scrutiny of birth and death records and any other age-related documents is necessary to support longevity claims. This type of centenarian validation in Loma Linda has not been reported. But what has been studied is the average longevity of California Seventh-day Adventists.

Californian Seventh-day Adventist Study – Gary Fraser is a Professor of Cardiology at the University of Loma Linda with an interest in the longevity of Seventh-day Adventists. Professor Fraser led a study of 34,192 Californian Seventh-day Adventists from 1975 to 1988[160,161]. In order to qualify for the study participants had to be white, non-Hispanic, at least 30 years old, and living in a California Adventist household. Sixty percent of those who qualified completed an extensive lifestyle questionnaire regarding their medical history, diet, physical activity, smoking habit, and a few psychosocial variables. In order to evaluate possible errors arising from the optical mark scanner and check for reliability of response 165 households (248 persons) were visited for a face-to-face interview. Subjects were contacted by mail every year to report any hospitalizations. Field staff visited hospitals and photocopied the subject's medical records that provided evidence of cardiovascular events or cancer. Mortality for all subjects was ascertained by matching to state death tapes and the National Death Index.

The study concluded that California Adventists, including those living in Loma Linda, have a higher life expectancy at the age of 30 than do other white Californians. Adventist's life expectancy was 7.3 years longer for men and 4.4 years longer for women than for other white California men and women[161]. A key to unlocking the secret of why Adventists live longer goes back to the founding tenants of their religion. A fundamental belief requires all members to abstain from any form of alcohol and tobacco. Possibly even more importantly, cofounder Ellen G. White prescribed drinking six to eight glasses of water a day. Water has always been believed to have the ability to flush toxins from the body, make the blood flow more freely, and prevent clotting. In addition, drinking six to eight glasses of water a day likely pushes both sugar sweetened and alcoholic beverages out of the diet.

Analysis of the data from the Californian Adventist study including a six-year follow-up revealed that among the 8,280 males and 12,017 females, who were without heart disease, stroke, and diabetes in 1976, there had been 246 fatal coronary heart disease events. Drinking five or more glasses of water a day was associated with a 54% less risk for men and a 41% less risk for women of fatal coronary heart disease compared with Adventists who drank only two glasses or less of water a day[160]. Even more dramatically, a high versus low intake of fluids other than water increased the risk to 146% in men and 247% in women[162]. A likely explanation for these results is that by adhering to Adventist's teachings both aluminum and ethanol in fluids other than water are prevented from inhibiting the detoxification of homocysteine that is a causal factor of atherosclerosis and heart disease[1]:

- Drinking more water means more OSA is consumed resulting in both more aluminum being excreted and more homocysteine being detoxified, lowering the risk of atherosclerosis and heart disease[1].
- Avoiding alcoholic beverages keeps plasma homocysteine at 8.5 to 9μM/L, decreasing the risk of atherosclerosis and heart disease[163].

Approximately 30% of those that participated in the Adventist study were vegetarians who ate meat less frequently than once a month and 23% ate nuts at least 5 times a week. The data from the Adventists study is compared with 1990 statistics on Japan and the U.S.A. in Table 17[161,164].

Table 17. Average Life Expectancy (LE) at Birth in Years[161,164]			
		Men	Women
Location	Years	LE From Birth (yr.)	LE From Birth (yr.)
California Adventists Vegetarians	1980-88	80.2	84.8
All Californian Adventists	1980-88	78.5	82.3
Japan	1990	75.9	81.8
U.S.A.	1990	73	79.6

Californian Adventists who are vegetarians have the longest life expectancy from birth when compared with all Californian Adventists and both Japan and the U.S.A. as shown in Table 17. Likely reasons for this are:

- Some vegetables are rich in OSA as they sequester OSA for aluminum toxicity protection[1]
- High vegetable protein diet with high levels of folic acid decreases homocysteine[165]

The difference between vegetarian and non-vegetarian Adventists extends to the risk of colon, prostate, and breast cancer as shown in Table 18[166]. This data for prostate and breast cancer mirrors the lower rates of these cancers in Okinawa versus mainland Japan (see Table 5).

Table 18. Relative Risk (RR) of Cancers in Vegetarian and Non-vegetarian Adventists[166]			
Cancer	Number of Cases	RR Vegetarians	RR Non-vegetarians
Colon	107	1.00	1.88
Prostate	127	1.00	1.54
Breast	128	1.00	1.25

Breast, prostate, and colon cancers have been linked to mutation in germ cells (i.e., cells when fully developed become sperm and ovum) of the *BRCA1* gene that prevent DNA repair by the BRCA1 protein[111]. *BRCA1* mutations are linked to 5-fold increased risk of colorectal cancers in women younger than 50 years of age[167]. Breast cancer has also been linked to decreased expression of the *BRCA1*gene[110]. Aluminum is a likely causal factor of these three cancers because it inhibits the expression of the *BRCA1* gene preventing DNA repair by the BRCA1 protein[110]. The lower rates of these cancers shown in Table 18 are likely due to both drinking more water containing OSA and eating more vegetables containing OSA. Some vegetables are good sources of OSA that may prevent the development of breast, prostate, and colon cancer by facilitating excretion of aluminum[1,165]. For information on OSA in vegetables see Chapter 4.

Approximately 40% of those that participated in the Adventist Health Study exercise vigorously for at least 15 minutes 3 times a week. Being more physically active in middle age extends life an extra 2.5 years[168]. Higher physical activity throughout life is estimated to extend life by 2.1 years[169]. Women who participated in the Adventist Health Study and exercised only infrequently had a 27% higher lifetime risk of breast cancer and an age of diagnosis of breast cancer 6 years younger on average than women who exercised frequently[170]. There are several reasons for this as described in my book Prevent Alzheimer's, Autism, and Stroke[1] but possibly the most important reason is that OSA in perspiration facilitates the excretion of aluminum in sweat (see Table 3)[74,75].

Loma Linda Drinking Water - Loma Linda gets its drinking water from three Mountain View Wells (3,5,6) and four Richardson Wells (3,4,5,6) that pump water out of the Bunker Hill Basin Aquifer. This aquifer extends from the San Bernardino Mountain Range to the south hills of Loma Linda. The water that replenishes the aquifer comes from rainfall and snowmelt from the San Bernardino Mountains. The wells are located in North Loma Linda. Loma Linda also uses supplemental water as needed from the City of San Bernardino Municipal Water Department[171].

The California Seventh-day Adventist Study was performed between 1975 and 1988 with a six-year follow-up in 1994. Just after the study and during the follow-up period in 1989 an appraisal of ground water quality in the Bunker Hill Basin was performed by the U.S. Geological Survey in cooperation with the San Bernardino Valley Municipal Water District[5]. Seven wells in North Loma Linda were tested for organics and inorganics including silica. The locations and number of the wells tested are indicated in Figure 20.

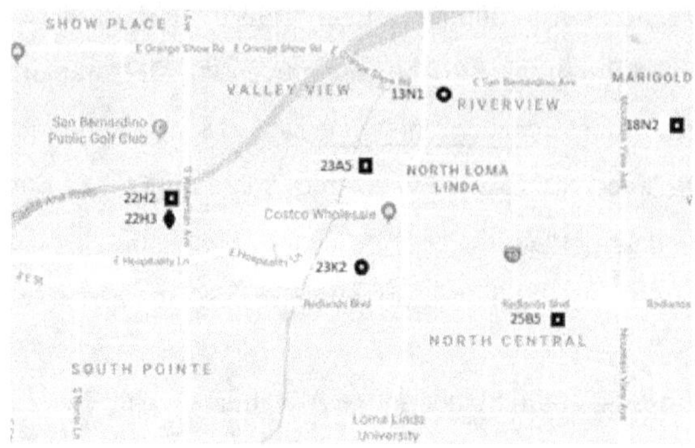

Figure 20. Seven wells in North Loma Linda: squares are lower aquifer, circles are upper aquifer, and diamond is lower and upper aquifer[5]

There are at least two aquifers, an upper and lower, under the area of the seven wells in North Loma Linda. These layers reach maximum depth and thickness in an underground canon along the Loma Linda Fault that runs on a straight line from the northwest to the southeast directly under well 23K2. Between half a mile southwest to two miles northeast of the Loma Linda Fault the upper aquifer is approximately 300 feet thick and the lower aquifer is approximately 600 feet thick. All seven of the wells tested are located above this underground canon[5].

The upper aquifer has water with slightly higher levels of OSA at 37ppm on average than the lower aquifer with 30ppm on average. Not surprisingly, the well that takes water from both aquifers is in the middle of the OSA range at 33.6ppm[5]. This data is summarized in Table 19 with reference to specific wells.

Table 19. OSA in Drinking Water from Seven Wells in North Loma Linda[5]		
Aquifer	**Well Number**	**OSA (ppm)**
Upper	23K2	38.4
Upper	13N1	35.2
Lower	25B5	35.2
Lower	23A5	33.6
Lower	18N2	25.6
Lower	22H2	25.6
Upper & Lower	22H3	33.6
		Avg. 32.5

For those of Loma Linda who follow the Adventists teachings and daily drink 6 to 8 glasses of water, they are effectively consuming the equivalent amount of OSA as someone who drinks 3 to

4 glasses of silica water containing 65ppm of OSA. In 2015 the amount of aluminum in Loma Linda's drinking water was 7.5ppb. Adventists in Loma Linda consume drinking water that is high in silica and low in aluminum and this may well be a causal factor for their longevity.

U.S.A. Drinking Water - In drinking water surveys of the large cities in the U.S.A., OSA was reported to vary from 0 to 115ppm with 11ppm as the median[3]. Raw waters in the U.S.A. may contain 1 to 48ppm of OSA[3]. Aluminum levels in U.S.A. drinking water are summarized in Table 20[3]. In the U.S.A. alum (a.k.a. aluminum sulfate) is the most common surface water treatment used. As indicted in Table 20 over half the alum treated drinking water in the U.S.A. contains over 100 ppb of aluminum. In the seven largest epidemiology studies to date, aluminum over 100 ppb has been linked to an elevated risk of Alzheimer's disease[1].

In order to lower aluminum in drinking water, treating with an iron coagulant versus an aluminum coagulant would be preferred as shown in Table 20[3]. Treating with iron does remove some silica from the water[3]. Most U.S.A. drinking waters need more silica added for the health of the population. Therefore, after treating surface water with iron, the water should be fortified with added dissolvable silica. All ground water that is low in silica should also be fortified.

Table 20. Aluminum levels in U.S. Raw and Finished Drinking Water[3]			
Water	**Coagulant**	**Aluminum Range (ppb)**	**Median Aluminum (ppb)**
Ground Water	None	14 - 290	31
Surface Water	None	16 – 1,167	43
Surface Water	Alum Coagulant	14 – 2,670	112
Surface Water	Iron Coagulant	15 - 81	38

Conclusion of Loma Linda Longevity Region - Loma Linda, like Okinawa, has shown us that reducing the body-burden of aluminum by drinking silica water can lower the risk of cardiovascular disease and cancer and increase longevity. The Adventists of California have demonstrated that drinking more water (greater than 5 glasses a day) does lower the risk of cardiovascular disease. The Adventists of Loma Linda who follow the teachings of the Ellen G.

White and drink 6 to 8 glasses of water a day, drink the equivalent of 3 to 4 glasses of 65ppm of OSA enriched water containing 15ppb of aluminum. This is in sharp contrast with the average drinking water in the U.S.A. with median levels of 11ppm OSA and 31ppb aluminum in ground water and 112ppb aluminum in treated surface water.

Also, the Adventist Health Study found that frequent exercise for at least 15 minutes 3 times a week can decrease both the risk of breast cancer and the age of diagnosis of breast cancer by 6 years. This translates to a life extension of 2.1 to 2.5 years and is likely due to OSA in perspiration facilitating the removal of aluminum from the body during exercise.

Adventists who are vegetarians have an increased amount of dietary OSA due to high levels of OSA in vegetables. Adventists who are gardeners in Loma Linda are enriching their vegetables with OSA due to irrigation with OSA rich tap water. This translates to a lower risk of cardiovascular disease and cancer resulting in a 1.7 to 2.5-year life extension.

West Hechi, China

Hechi is a prefecture located in the north of the Guangxi region of China (see Figure 21). The Guangxi region is in southern China on the border with Viet Nam. In western Hechi there are three adjacent counties with much higher centenarian prevalences and longevity indexes than three adjacent counties to the east in central Hechi. The longevity counties are: Bama Yao, Fengshan, and Donglan with Bama Yao being a super longevity region having the highest longevity index. The non-longevity counties are: Huanjiang, Jinchengjiang, and Nandan. The Duyang Mountains separate the longevity counties from the non-longevity counties (see Figure 21).

Bama Yao Longevity Region Verification – In 1992 Yang used data from the 1990 census and from a questionnaire survey conducted in Bama Yao to analyze the population age 80 and over[462]. In May to June of 1994 three Chinese demographers evaluated the quality of Yang's survey data by interviewing 67 out of 73 people over age 100 in Bama Yao[463]. Age records were available from birth registers and generation rankings. They found that only 3 centenarians still had spouses and 42 were women and 25 were men. The people of Bama Yao are comprised of 13 ethnic groups with only 17.4% being Yao. The demographers found Yang's survey data to be reliable.

Air Quality in Bama Yao - The centenarian prevalence and the longevity index of 31 regions in China, including Guangxi, were evaluated in 2016 with respect to air quality parameters[464]. Sulfur dioxide and particulates in the air, 10nm or smaller, were negatively correlated with centenarian prevalence and the longevity index, respectively. The three longevity counties and three non-longevity counties in Guangxi, including Bama Yao, are located in remote mountainous areas (see Figure 21) and therefore their air quality is well above average. **Because all six counties have the same air quality, it is not possible that air quality is a factor in the observed longevity in Bama Yao.**

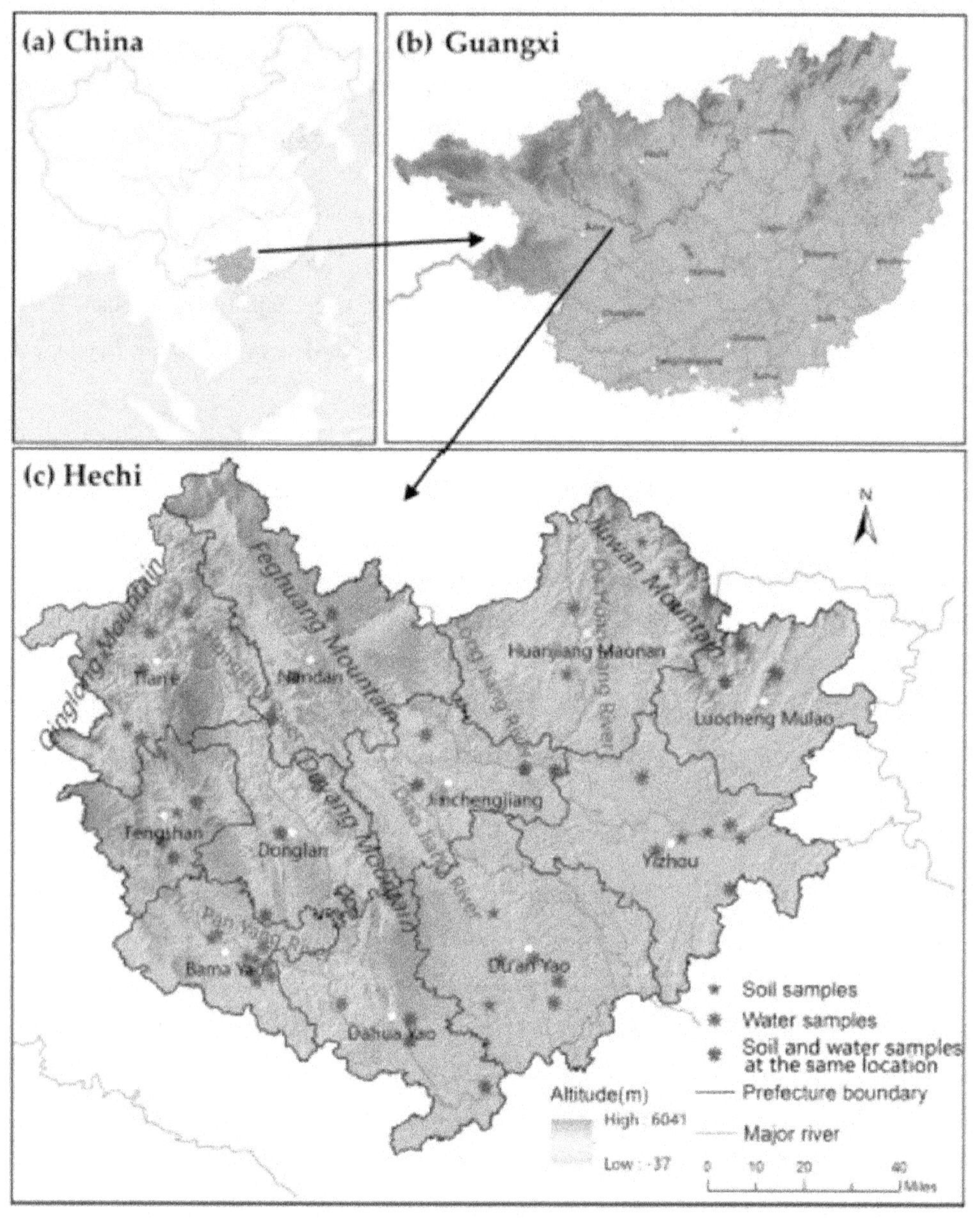

Figure 21 – Location of Hechi and its sampling sites (c) in Gurangxi (b), China (a) [461]

Natural and Socioeconomic Factors in Bama Yao – Natural factors, such as temperature and altitude, and socioeconomic factors, such as gross domestic product (a.k.a. GDP) , economic status, education, local infrastructure, and health care facilities, were evaluated spatially and geographically with respect to 7 longevity indicators, including centenarian prevalence and longevity index, in 109 selected counties and districts in Guangxi[465]. The results indicated only a weak association with longevity and natural factors, such as temperature and altitude, and socioeconomic factors, such as GDP per capita. However, the average GDP in Hechi was comparatively lower than other regions in Guangxi[461].   All the longevity and non-longevity counties in West Hechi have similar topography and temperatures. **Therefore, there is no natural of socioeconomic factor that stands out as being a contributor to the longevity observed in Bama Yao.**

Environmental Factors in Bama Yao – Trace elements in the soil and drinking water of Hechi were evaluated temporally and spatially with respect to centenarian prevalence and longevity index from 1982 to 2010[461]. The trace elements measured in the drinking water sampled from 40 locations were: Pb, Zn, Cd, SO_4^{2-}, Mn, **H_2SiO_3**, Ca, Fe, Na, Mg, Li, Mo, and Se. The trace elements measured in soil were: Sr, K, Mo, Fe, Co, Zn, Cu. **The only trace element in soil and drinking water that showed a significant (0.01 level) positive correlation with both centenarian prevalence and longevity index is H_2SiO_3. This trace element forms a hydrate in water called OSA (H_4SiO_4). For details see Table 4 at the beginning of this chapter.**

The following paragraph is taken from the paper linking OSA to longevity in the three longevity counties, including Bama Yao[461]: "As many centenarians live in rocky areas[466], most of the members of the longevity population in Hechi use the underground water source as their primary water supply. These areas do not have much surface water but do have abundant quantities of underground water from underground caverns. For example, in 1982, 1990, and 2000, approximately 75% of the centenarians in Bama County lived in rocky and semi-rocky areas and used underground water as their main water source, and approximately 30% of the underground water areas have sustained approximately 70% of the centenarians in Bama over decades[467]. It can be inferred that the distinctive tectonic settings of Hechi might have long-term impacts on longevity in this region".

Distinctive Tectonic Setting of West Hechi, China

The tectonic setting of western Guangxi has been studied[468]. The Duyang Mountains that separate the longevity from the non-longevity counties in Hechi lie along a geological rift. Rifts occur linearly along the central axis of most mid-ocean ridges where two tectonic plates are diverging and literally pulling apart the earth's crust. The result is a long wide valley to the west of the Duyang Mountains where the three longevity counties are located called the Danchi Rift Trough[468]. This area is distinctive because drinking water in this area is significantly higher in OSA than the area just to the east of the Duyang Mountains[461].

Deep-water ocean sediments from the late Early Devonian to the late Permian have been uplifted in the Danchi Rift Trough. The chert that underlies Bama Yao is from the Middle Permian period[469]. The rocks in this area are mostly chert containing greater than 70% silicon dioxide (SiO_2) derived from non-terrigenous (i.e., marine) sediments[468]. Sources of these marine sediments can be of either biogenic or hydrothermal origin.

The source of silica in this chert is predominantly biogenic being derived from siliceous organisms such as radiolarians, diatoms, and siliceous sponges[468]. This chert is richer in SiO_2 than modern oceanic siliceous sediment and less rich in SiO_2 as compared with the nearly pure SiO_2 in chert from terrigenous sources, such as volcanos[468]. Enrichment of biogenic SiO_2 in chert is hypothesized to occur by a process called diagenetic silicification that more than doubles the SiO_2 in chert[470]. In this process water enriched in OSA displaces calcium carbonate in chert making biogenic SiO_2 (a.k.a. opal)[471].

Opal is a good source of OSA as it is the most soluble solid silicate in sediments[472]. When water comes in contact with different types of opal sediments at pore depths greater than 10cm the equilibrium concentration of OSA in the water is from 9.6 to 72ppm (100 to 750mcM L^{-1})[472]. **The unique conditions required for diagenetic silicification resulting in opal deposits may account for the unique OSA rich well water found in the Danchi Rift Trough in West Hetchi, China.**

Marion, Iowa

Driven by the increasing cost of caring for the elderly population in the U.SA., states are looking at health initiatives led by communities and businesses. These grassroots efforts are promoted by political leaders with the goals of increasing their state's health ranking and saving money on health care. An example is Iowa where on August 10th 2011 Governor Terry Bradstad challenged fellow Iowans to make the Hawkeye State the healthiest state in the nation by 2016. In 2011 Iowa was ranked the 19th most healthy state in the union. The Governor proposed in his Healthiest State Initiative that if Iowan's adopted some lifestyle changes, their quality of life could be improved while saving the state $18 billion in costs for caring for the elderly over the 5-year period from 2011 to 2016.

One of these 10 Iowa cities selected for this initiative was Marion, where my father lived for his entire life, except for the six years he spent in the navy during World War II. My mother lived in their single-family home in Marion until she was 94½ the last 2½ years by herself after my father died in 2019 at age 95. My mother and father both decided in 2014 to change the quality of their lives by daily drinking silica rich water. This lifestyle change continued for 5 years and resulted in my mother's memory improving sufficiently to continue living in her home needing minimal medical and caretaking support. My mother is an example of healthy longevity that can cut the costs for caring for the elderly.

Marion Drinking Water - The drinking water in Marion comes from the Jordan aquafer that underlies most of Iowa. The OSA concentration in the aquifer is reported to vary from 8 to 48ppm (5-30ppm SiO_2) [171]. Unfortunately, Marion is located in the area of 13ppm OSA (8ppm SiO_2) or less[173]. In 2018 the measured concentration of OSA in Marion tap water was only 2ppm[174].

Conclusion of Marion, Iowa - My mom had been diagnosed with cognitive impairment in 2012 that was impacting her daily living skills. Because of this in 2012 I began researching preventative treatments for Alzheimer's disease. By 2014 I recommended my parents daily drink 3 to 4 cups of Fiji water containing approximately 124ppm of OSA[174,175]. Fiji water is available at the local grocery store but it was very heavy to lug home. Amazon Prime came to the rescue with free delivery of Fiji water to my parent's door at a price lower than the grocery store's price. If Marion added silica to their drinking water, the entire city would stand an excellent chance of becoming a longevity region.

I am delighted to say that when I began my research into why my mother's short-term memory was failing, she mostly talked about things that happened 60 years ago. Now every time we talk, she describes in detail things that have happened during the day and in the last few days. While daily drinking silica rich water my mother's cognition continued to improve as demonstrated by two mini-mental state examinations (a.k.a. MMSE) administered by her doctor. She scored 22 out of 30 in September of 2017 and scored 24 out of 30 in September of 2018 with scores of 20 to 24 being regarded as mild cognitive impairment (a.k.a. MCI).

I primarily attribute her Alzheimer's reversal to drinking silica rich water. In addition, she has followed the recommendations of my first book, including frequent physical activity with some perspiration[1]. I can only hope that others will follow in my mother's footsteps and drink silica rich water, change their lifestyle choices, and take the several daily supplements I recommend[1]. Why wait for a promised cure when you can take action now while you still have your mental health.

Conclusion of Silica Water for Healthy Longevity

Loren Eiseley was correct when he said "If there is magic on this planet, it is in the water." The magic is called dissolved silica as OSA and it is the secret of healthy longevity. It is indeed remarkable that a common thread has been found to exist in all six longevity regions. That common thread is OSA enriched silica drinking water.

We must thank the demographers who identified the six longevity regions as they have given us the chance to explore the magic and understand the secret of why the people of these regions have extreme longevity. This exploration has opened our eyes to OSA in drinking water as a naturally occurring safe and inexpensive preventative for common fatal diseases, such as cardiovascular disease, cancer, and Alzheimer's. Drinking more silica water than normal allows some Seventh-day Adventists, who follow the teachings of the church, to double the amount of OSA they consume. This may account for why Adventists who drank five or more glasses of silica water a day had a 54% less risk for men and a 41% less risk for women of a fatal coronary heart disease event compared with Adventists who drank only two glasses or less of silica water a day[160].

Because OSA rich silica water both facilitates the elimination of aluminum from the body and lowers the risk of common fatal diseases, such as cardiovascular, cancer, and Alzheimer's, it further implicates aluminum as a causal factor of these diseases. The finding that people who migrate out of Nicoya do not have the extreme life expectancy of those that have spent their life in Nicoya supports the contention that Nicoya's longevity is due to an environmental factor, such as OSA rich silica water, and not genetics.

Physical movement or exercise is commonly performed in all longevity regions. For instance, in Ikaria, 89% of men and 70% of women performed moderate to high daily physical activity and only 0.8% of men and 0.3% of women owned a car. This is typical of longevity regions since their populations are at the low end of the economic spectrum, with the exception of Loma Linda. Also, longevity regions are in general hilly areas requiring additional effort to move about. Physical exercise is good for a number of reasons[1], but possibly most importantly it results in perspiration. Aluminum is excreted in perspiration and OSA facilitates this by increasing the concentration of aluminum excreted in the sweat of men and women[74,75]. This may account for why Seventh-day Adventist women who exercised only infrequently had a 27% higher lifetime risk of breast cancer and an age of diagnosis of breast cancer 6 years younger on average than Adventist women who exercised frequently[170].

There are unexpected differences between men and women centenarians in longevity regions. For instance, in Okinawa the ratio of female to male centenarians is 5 to 1 while in Villagrande it is 1 to 1. The Okinawan centenarians did not drink OSA rich silica water until 1933 to 1944 and then after 1951 when their water supply was rebuilt after World War II. Those living in Villagrande benefitted from OSA rich silica water from conception to at least 1949 when Lago Bau Muggens was created. Therefore, OSA in drinking water from conception seems to benefit the life expectancy of young men more than young women and could account for Villagrande's unique 1 to 1 female to male ratio of centenarians not seen in the Okinawan longevity region.

Evolutionarily men have evolved to not only produce more sweat by volume than women but when drinking OSA rich silica water, men's sweat has a higher concentration of aluminum than women's sweat. This evolutionary advantage for men could be the reason OSA rich silica water benefits men more than women. This may be either in spite of or an evolutionary response to boys absorbing more aluminum than girls.

As Benjamin Franklin pointed out in 1736 "an ounce of prevention is worth a pound of cure". States and their communities are beginning to embrace this as witnessed in Iowa where a grass roots effort to lower health care costs by improving community health was implemented in 2013. In the 5-year time period between 2013 and 2018 Iowa's ranking was raised from 19th to the 13th most healthy state in the union. In order to achieve even greater success in Iowa at least 50ppm of OSA should be added to community drinking water. Only by making OSA rich silica water available to all, will we have true-blue longevity regions.

Another common thread that exists in all longevity regions is OSA rich vegetables in the diet. This diet has been called the Mediterranean Diet. The fact that vegetarians live longer than non-vegetarians is not surprising, as vegetables sequester OSA for their own protection against aluminum in the soil. Vegetables are a supplementary source of OSA in the diet as discussed in the next chapter.

Chapter 4 – Dietary Bioavailable Dissolved Silica

In addition to silica in drinking water being at abnormally high levels in all longevity regions, another common factor is the above normal amount of home or locally grown vegetables consumed in longevity regions. As described in Chapter 2 vegetables sequester silica for defense against aluminum. Eating a vegetable with sequestered OSA involves transferring the defense from vegetables to humans. Therefore, just like drinking OSA rich silica water, eating OSA rich vegetables promotes longevity by lowering the risk of three common fatal diseases:

- **Cancer** - Vegetarians have a significantly lower risk of breast, prostate, and colon cancer than non-vegetarians[166].
- **Dementia** – Non-Vegetarians in California have twice the risk of having dementia as compared with vegetarians, except in Loma Linda[176]. This exception could be explained simply as both non-vegetarians and vegetarians in Loma Linda get high levels of OSA from their drinking water and therefore both have a lower risk of dementia.
- **Cardiovascular Disease** – People who took part in the Nurse's Health Study (75,600 women and 38,700 men) who were in the highest quintile of fruit and vegetable intake had 31% lower risk of ischemic stroke and 20% lower risk of coronary heart disease[177,178]. This translates to a 6% lower risk of stroke and a 4% lower risk of coronary heart disease for every daily serving of fruits or vegetables[177,178].

These are the same three diseases that are found to be lower in longevity regions of Okinawa and Loma Linda. Also, Ikarians have approximately 20% lower rates of cancer, 50% lower rates of heart disease, and 25% less dementia[137]. In addition, the Nicoyan advantage comes primarily from lower male cardiovascular mortality[136,149]. Although OSA in longevity region drinking water may be the primary reason for low rates of these terminal diseases, an important secondary factor is the consumption in longevity regions of home or locally grown garden vegetables biofortified with irrigation water containing more silica than normal.

The advantage of eating vegetables at the expense of meat works best if the vegetables are rich in silica. In longevity regions where drinking water and irrigation water come from the same silica rich sources, there is an enhancement of silica in vegetables by fertilization with silica water. Irrigation of crops with silica enriched (50 to 100ppm) water has been shown to increase the silica biofortification of leafy vegetables with an increase silica bioavailability in the edible parts as shown in Table 21[179].

Fruits, such as apples, bananas, and grapes, can also be enriched in silica with application of silica fertilizer[180-182]. In the case of grapes, fertilizing with 112ppm OSA resulted in 20% more accumulation of silica in the leaves of some cultivars[182]. Analysis of the leaves of these fertilized grapes revealed 2% (20,000mg/Kg) total silica (SiO_2) by weight and 0.1% by (1,000mg/Kg) weight of water soluble OSA. This is significant because grape wine and leaves are a part of the diet in the Mediterranean longevity regions.

Table 21. Biofortication of Leafy Vegetable with Silica Enriched Irrigation Water[179]			
Leafy Vegetable	**No Silica Enrichment SiO_2 Content mg/Kg**	**With 50–100ppm Silica SiO_2 Content mg/Kg**	**% Enhancement**
Basil	41	294	617
Chicory	23	76	230
Mizuna	19	106	458
Purslane	15	93	520
Swiss Chard	17	76	347
Tatsoi	18	69	283

The beneficial silica in vegetables and fruit is in two forms: water soluble OSA and water insoluble biosilifications of SiO_2, such as phytoliths. OSA lowers aluminum absorption in the gut and reverses aluminum accumulation in the body as shown in Table 1[64]. Oligomeric (i.e., polymeric) silica has an affinity for aluminum in the gut that surpasses even OSA[30]. For this reason, it is not surprising that phytoliths also have an affinity for aluminum forming HAS on their surfaces[58]. The more HAS coating the surfaces of phytoliths, the less they dissolve as OSA in water[184]. When phytoliths are ingested they lower aluminum absorption in the gut and enhance aluminum excretion. Therefore, eating vegetables and fruit provides humans with two forms of beneficial silica: OSA for lowering accumulated aluminum in the body and both OSA and biosilifactions of SiO_2 for decreasing aluminum absorption in the gut.

Declining Sources of Silica in the Diet

Because of silica's abundance in the earth's crust most soils formerly contained sufficient silica to allow plants grown on this soil to maximize their silica accumulation[185]. However, after many years of harvesting crops and only fertilizing with phosphorus, nitrogen, and potassium, both the soil upon which these crops are grown and the crops themselves have become nutrient depleted[186]. The vegetables and fruits we eat today are silica deficient compared with those eaten by our ancestors.

There are plants that accumulate silica at concentrations of over 1% by weight and accumulate more silica than calcium[185]. Eight of the 10 most produced crops of the world are silica accumulators and all 9 of the most produced crops in the U.S.A. are silica accumulators as listed in Table 22[187,188]. In the U.S.A. production of these 9 crops removes approximately 10 million tons of silicon that is equivalent to 34 million tons of OSA from the soil each year. The OSA removal rate from the entire U.S.A. cropland is estimated at approximately twice this level annually[187]. Without the application of silica fertilizers, the silica in the food we eat has declined and will continue decline. For this reason, supplementing our drinking water with OSA rich silica water makes good sense.

Table 22. Estimated Shoot Silicon Uptake Worldwide and in the U.S. from 2004 to 2013[187,188]				
Crops	World Production Million Tons	U.S. Production Million Tons	% Si in Shoots	Annual U.S. Si Uptake in Tons
Sugar Cane	1,736	27.4	1.5	58,000
Maize	826	307.8	0.8-1.4	4,210,000
Rice	686	9.5	4.2	395,000
Wheat	683	58.4	2.5	2,144,000
Potatoes	326		0.4	
Cassava	232		0.5	
Soybeans	231	84.7	1.4	1,766,000
Sugar Beet	222	29.2	2.3	683,000
Barley	155	4.6	1.8	126,000
Tomatoes	136		1.6	
Oats		1.3	1.5	27,000
Sorghum		9.3	1.5	144,000
Total				9,552,000

Worldwide two of the largest silicon accumulator crops are sugar cane and rice as shown in Table 22. Magnesium silicate used as a fertilizer resulted in the yield of sugar cane in the Cauca Valley of Columbia increasing by 14.6% and sugar production increased by 20%. Likewise, rice production in the Magdalena Valley and Atlantic coastal areas of Columbia increased by 21% to 33%[189]. This work shows that using silica fertilizers can financially help farmers by improving crop yield while at the same time improving the health and longevity of crop consumers.

The use of magnesium and calcium silicates as fertilizer has an even greater benefit than improving human health, longevity, and crop yield: it removes carbon dioxide (CO_2) from the atmosphere **slowing global warming**[480]. The following two reactions summarize the natural weathering of rocks, such as olivine (Mg_2SiO_4) and wollastonite ($CaSiO_3$):

- $Mg_2SiO_4 + 4\ CO_2 + 4\ H_2O\ \rightarrow\ 2\ Mg^{++} + 4HCO_3^- + H_4SiO_4$ (OSA)
- $CaSiO_3 + CO_2 + 2\ H_2O\ \rightarrow\ Ca^{++} + CO_3^{-2} + H_4SiO_4$ (OSA)

Both the weathering and fertilization processes are enhanced with natural soil organisms and by milling the rock to increase its surface area[480]. The carbonate (CO_3^{-2}) and bicarbonate (HCO_3^-) neutralize the soil by counteracting acid rain and ultimately, when dissolved in rain water runoff, will counteract ocean acidification, an effect of rising CO_2[480]. The OSA formed by these reactions fertilizes the soil improving crop yield and the health and longevity of crop consumers.

Current Sources of Silica in the Diet

Silica from plants comes primarily from grains, vegetables, fruit, and products of grains and fruit, such as beer and wine. Foods made from these plant sources make up what is called the Mediterranean Diet that is a common thread of all six longevity regions. Table 23 provides guidance on which foods have more silica content[79,190-193]. Note that high silica content does not necessarily mean that the silica is dissolvable, absorbed, and therefore bioavailable. The numbers in parenthesis are the percentage of absorbed and bioavailable silica in 100 grams of food[79,191-193]. Foods too low in silica to be in this table include nuts, milk, milk products, meat, and meat products[79,191-193].

Table 23. Silicon Content of Food[79,190-193]		
Food (100 grams)	**Silicon Content (milligrams)**	**Silicon Absorbed as OSA (percent)**
Oats (including husks/hulls)	278	49
Cassava Root (fermented with skin)	270	?
Barley	109	49
Potatoes (including skin)	93	21
Whole Wheat Grain	74	?
Oat Bran	23	49
Dates (dried)	16.6	17
Granola Cereals	12.2	49
Porridge (processed dry oats)	11.4	49
Wheat Bran Cereal (high fiber)	10-11.4	49
Red Beets	9.3	21
Asparagus	8.4	21
Raisins (California seedless)	8.2	44
Spinach (fresh – boiled)	5.1	?
Bananas (peeled)	4.77-5.4	4
Lentils (red, boiled)	4.42	?
Pineapple (fresh and canned)	3.93-4.53	?
Cucumber/Bitter Melon (fresh, raw)	2.53	?
Green Beans (boiled)	2.4-8.73	44
Whole Grain Bread	2.3 – 4.78	49
Carrots & Parsnips (raw, peeled, boiled)	2.3	26
Brown Rice (boiled with husks)	2.1-3.76	41
Corn (flakes, chips, and tortillas)	1.9-4.4	49
Spring Greens	1.81	?
Beer (filtered alcoholic/non-alcoholic)	0.9-3.94	56-60
Whole Grain Pasta	1.29	?
Wine – Red, White, Port, Sherry, Rose	0.68-2.31	?
Avocados (fresh without skin and stone)	0.64	?
Grapes – Green and Red	0.49	?
Potato (white or sweet: peeled or boiled)	0.27-0.55	21
Raw Fruit	0.1-2.5	?

Fluids account for 20 to 30% of our dietary intake of OSA and the ingestion of solid foods account for the rest. In order for OSA to be absorbed from solid foods these foods must be hydrolyzed in the acidity of our gastrointestinal (GI) tract. Since the kidney is the major route for silica excretion, urinary silicon levels are an indicator of silica absorption and bioavailability.

A semi-quantitative study was performed measuring the dietary intake of silica in foods eaten by members of the Framingham study[192]. A 126-item food frequency questionnaire was filled out to get a measure of what is consumed on average by members of the study. A second part of the study involved overnight fasting of healthy volunteers followed by ingestion of a test meal and then 6 more hours of fasting. Throughout this period of time the volunteers only drank ultra-high purity water containing negligible silicon content. Urine samples were taken and analyzed for silicon as a measure of silica absorption and bioavailability. The results indicated that between 13 and 62mg/day of silicon was ingested per day and 43% of this silicon was absorbed and bioavailable as dissolved silica (OSA). The major food sources for silica among women were bananas and string beans accounting for 17% of dietary silica intake. The major food sources for silica among men were beer and bananas accounting for 25% of dietary silica intake. Women in this study have less bioavailable silica than men because men consume more beer than women. For children in this study the major dietary source of silica is from cereals (68% of total dietary intake).

Most of the silicon in the grains, vegetables, and fruit we eat is in the husks, hulls, and skin. Processed foods have the silica rich husks, hulls, and skins removed thereby lowering their silica levels. Because of minimal processing our paleo hunter gatherer ancestors had a diet much richer in silica than our modern diet. Note from the box plot in Figure 8 that as we age our serum silicon levels decline[85]. Intake of silica decreases with age in humans declining at a rate of 100μg/year of age after age 39[192,193]. This decline in intake of silica at least partially accounts for why aluminum absorption in humans increases with age[194] resulting in an increased rate of aluminum accumulation in elderly (75-101 years of age) versus non-elderly human brains[195].

Therefore, I recommend OSA supplementation particularly as you age and when you are pregnant and breast feeding.

Dietary Silica for Longevity

We have linked dissolved silica in water (i.e., OSA) to longevity in Chapter 3 and in this chapter we have so far linked good health to eating grain, vegetables, and fruit high in bioavailable silica. But does eating food high in bioavailable silica correlate with longevity? One factor that is common to all longevity regions is that they are populated primarily with people who eat unprocessed foods that contain more silica than processed foods. Examples taken from Table 23 include:

- Oats with husks and hulls contain 19 times more silica than processed dry oats used for porridge.
- Potatoes with skins contain 344 times more silica than potatoes peeled and boiled.
- Whole wheat grain contains 14 times more silica than high-fiber wheat bran cereal.

As testimony to longevity there is a family in Ireland named Donnelly that in 2017 had 13 living siblings with a total age of 1075 years. This family has been made famous by being named the oldest family in the world by the Guinness Book of World Records. When asked for the secret of their longevity, Leo Donnelly 72 the youngest sibling claims "We have always followed Daddy's habit of that nice warm bite before sleep - porridge at around 10PM, then porridge again for breakfast at 7AM - cooked oats, milk, and perhaps a spot of jam on top."[196] So is there something in the oat porridge that might be contributing to the Donnelly's longevity?

In Ireland and Scotland there is Celtic oat porridge called sowans (a.k.a. sowens, virpa) that has historically been very popular with the poor. Sowans is made from the husks (a.k.a. sids) containing some residual meal left over after the milling process of oats. This oat porridge was served both daily and traditionally on special occasions, such as Christmas Eve and/or Christmas morning. Sowans is made by steeping oat husks in water for one to seven days (the longer the more sour the product) and then straining out the undissolved husks. The strained liquid contains a fine flowery meal that is allowed to settle out during a day of "fermenting". This nutrient rich starchy solid matter is boiled in salted water and served as sowans. The liquid drained off after fermentation is called "sowan-swats" and used as a drink for children or substitute for milk in baking or in tea[197,198].

It is a safe-bet that sowan and sowan-swats contains very high levels of bioavailable silica. From Table 23 it can be calculated that a bowl of sowan made from 40 grams of oatmeal with husk and hulls could provide as much as 117mg of bioavailable silica. This is unlike a bowl of 40 grams of processed dry oats (i.e., porridge) that only provides 4.8mg of bioavailable silica.

So, what fruits and vegetables do people in longevity regions eat that could be adding silica to their diets? Here is a brief synopsis of his study with foods ranked by their silicon content in milligrams per 100gram serving[199]:

Okinawan Food

Sweet potatoes with skins (93mg Si/100gr): Since the 17th century a staple of the Okinawan diet has been the satsuma-imo a purple sweet potato. Also, its leaves are eaten as greens in miso soup. The satsuma-imo was introduced to Okinawa from the Americas about 400 years ago and took well to Okinawan soil. Before 1940 more than 60% of the calories consumed by Okinawans were from the satsuma-imo. The traditional diet was about 80 percent carbohydrates.

Bitter melon (2.5mg Si/100gr): Names can be deceiving as this melon is a vegetable and not a fruit. It looks like a type of cucumber and when green it can be bitter tasting. Usually, it is stir-fried with a medley of vegetables in a dish called goya champuru.

Brown rice boiled with husks (2.1-3.8mg Si/100gr): Okinawans eat both brown and white rice every day.

Comments About Okinawan Food: It is obvious based upon the relative amounts of silica in these vegetables that the satsuma-imo provided the bulk of the silica assuming the skin was eaten. But prior to the exponential increase in centenarians on Okinawa that occurred between 1974 and 2006 (see Figure 9) a fast-food invasion hit Okinawa. According to Japanese Government Surveys between 1949 and 1960 dietary calories derived from sweet potatoes declined from 60% to 5% and during this time rice consumption doubled and meat, eggs, and poultry consumption increased more than sevenfold[199,200]. Not coincidentally cancers of the lung, breast, and colon almost doubled by 1960[199,201].

Okinawa was occupied by the U.S.A. for 27 years, from the end of World War II until 1972. Despite of reversion back to Japanese rule, Okinawa still has a large presence of U.S.A. forces that has continued to shape the islands culinary preferences. In 1963 the fast-food chain A&W opened their first franchise outside of North America in Okinawa introducing root beer, hamburgers, and fries. This fast food quickly became popular and by 2015 there were 26 A&W locations on Okinawa[202]. Okinawa has 8.2 hamburger joints per 100,000 people, more than anywhere else in Japan[203]. The fast-food invasion became a fusion of local and western tastes. For instance, Blue Seal ice cream became available in Okinawa in 1948. This iconic U.S.A. brand comes in 30 flavors, including satsuma-imo sweet potato flavor but without the skin and silica[202].

Okinawan centenarians who were born around 1900 ingested high levels of OSA from two different sources during their lives. The satsuma-imo sweet potato provided most of the OSA during the first half of their lives and drinking water from the northern part of the island provided most of the OSA during the last quarter of their lives. Fast-foods containing less than 1% of the silicon content of the satsuma-imo sweet potato had a negative impact on Okinawan health from 1950 to 1974. However, after the Fukuji Reservoir began supplying drinking water to Okinawans in 1974, the rise in dissolved silica in drinking water fully compensated for the fast-food invasion by leading to an exponential increase in Okinawan centenarians.

Sardinian Food

Several researchers have looked back at what Sardinian's, who became centenarians from 1980 to 2000, ate from birth to middle age. Nutritional data from the 1930's was performed by both Italian hygienist C. Fermi and dietary researcher G. Peretti[199,204-206]. Fermi and Peretti found that in a month, adults living in the Sardinian hills consumed the following[199,204-206].

Potatoes with skins (93mg Si/100gr.): Sardinians consume potatoes as a major portion of their 84,000 calories per month.

Whole Grain Bread (2.3-4.8mg Si/100gr.): Wheat flour is made into 11 pounds of flat and sourdough bread a month. Barley flour is made into 4 pounds of barley bread (a.k.a. *orgiathu*) a month.

Red Wine (0.7mg Si/100gr): Sardinians drink 7 liters of Cannonau wine made from Grenache grapes in a month. Although viewed as important for longevity wine may be over rated based upon the fact that it contains less the 1% of the silica in barley and potatoes (see Table 23).

Comments About Sardinian Food: A factor in how the people living in Barbagia hill country of Sardinia prepare food is that they are some of the poorest people in Italy. It is likely that all parts of the grain and potato, including the hulls and skin, are prepared and eaten. In 1938 G. Peretti, surveyed 28 farming families and 17 shepherd families living in three Sardinian villages[199,206]. Peretti found that on a calorie basis the people consumed the following:

- Carbohydrates from potatoes, bread, pasta, and beans – 65%
- Fat from goat's milk, sheep's cheese, and olive oil – 20%
- Protein primarily from beans and occasionally sheep, pig, and chicken (never fish) – 15%

Sardinian centenarians have eaten during their lives a diet rich in silica due to potatoes, bread, pasta, and beans that in total provided 65% of their caloric intake. Fats and animal protein provided 35% of their caloric intake and these foods are very low in silica. Protein was never from fish as it was a two-day trip to the sea from the highlands.

Ikarian Food

Because of the island's isolation the population has adhered to an old dietary culture that has avoided western influence. The diet of Ikarians favors vegetables and whole grains and is based around the following foods with percentage of daily intake in grams[199]:

Potatoes with skins (93mg Si/100gr.): Boiled potatoes – 9%

Asparagus (18mg Si/100gr.): Plus vegetables from local gardens – 20%

Lentils (4.4mg Si/100gr.): Plus garbanzo beans and black-eyed peas - 11%

Whole Grain Bread (2.3-4.8mg Si/100gr.): Made into sourdough bread - ?%

Spring Greens (1.8mg Si/100gr.): As 150 varieties of wild greens grow on the island – 17%

Whole Grain Pasta (1.3mg Si/100gr.): - 5%

Red Wine (0.7mg Si/100gr): Ikarians drink a moderate amount of wine

Raw Fruit (0.1-2.5mg Si/100gr.): Lemons are used on everything and eaten with skin – 16%

Living on an island makes Ikarians careful to prepare and eat all parts of the grains and vegetables they grow. Eating skins and husks increases the amount of silica they ingest.

Nicoyan Food

The Nicoya peninsula is geographically isolated from mainland Costa Rica isolating its population from western culinary influence. In 1957 a Berkeley anthropologist by the name of Phillip Wagner wrote a report entitled "Nicoya: a Cultural Geography"[207]. In his report Wagner describes the traditional food eaten daily by Nicoya farmers. A staple is *gallo pinto* made by frying rice and beans in pork fat. This is eaten daily with corn (a.k.a. maize) tortillas and eggs. Soups are also made with plantains, taro, or yucca. Sketches of local gardens indicated more than 40 edible plant species are grown including: papaya, yam, and bananas. The Nicoya diet also includes a wide variety of forest fruits.

Dietary surveys indicate that 67% of the Nicoya diet is carbohydrates that include: vegetables 14%, fruits 9%, legumes 7%, grains 26%, sugars 11%, and with the non-carbohydrates being dairy 24% and protein-fat 9%[208]. The portion of the Nicoya diet that is highest in OSA is the following:

Yams unpeeled and boiled (93mg Si/100gr.): Because of the low socioeconomic status of Nicoyans, it is likely that yams are eaten unpeeled. Unrelated to North American sweet potatoes, the Nicoyan yam is firm and white even when cooked.

Yams peeled and boiled (0.37mg Si/100gr.): It is unlikely yams are peeled before cooking in Nicoya.

Bananas peeled (4.8-5.4mg Si/100gr.): They are a staple of Nicoya and eaten every day. These include plantains that do not sweeten as they ripen and are usually fried.

Corn Tortillas (1.9-4.4mg Si/100gr.): Nicoyans make corn (a.k.a. *maize nixamal or nixquezado*) tortillas and eat them as all three meals during the day. The corn is soaked in lime in order to release niacin, and then ground into flour.

Black-Eyed and Black Beans boiled (1.2mg Si/100gr.): Nicoyans eat black beans almost everyday

White Rice (1-2mg Si/100gr.): During the last 50 years white rice has replaced squash as a staple food of Nicoya

Plums (0.25mg Si/100gr.): Pejivalles are an oval orange colored plum that is a staple food for Nicoyans.

Raw Fruit (0.1-2.5mg Si/100gr.): Nicoyans eat one papaya daily.

Unpeeled yams are the major source of silica in the Nicoyan diet second only to Nicoyan drinking water (17-41mg Si/liter). Bananas and corn tortillas are also important sources of silica in the Nicoyan diet.

Adventist Food

Living in the U.S.A. it is hard to avoid fast food and prepared food that has been stripped of silica. The Adventist lifestyle promotes eating local grown fruits and vegetables as 70% of their caloric intake. The portion of the Adventist diet that is highest in OSA is the following:

Red Beets (21mg Si/100gr.): Seventy percent of the Adventist diet is fruits and vegetables.

Porridge made of processed dry oats (11.4mg Si/100gr.): Slow-cooked oatmeal is a staple for Adventists. Many Adventists who are centenarians say that oatmeal is their breakfast.

Potatoes without skins (0.3-0.6mg Si/100gr.): In the U.S.A. we generally peel potatoes prior to cooking. The skin of potatoes contains almost all of the silica (see Table 23).

Cucumbers (2.5mg Si/100gr.): Served and eaten fresh and raw with skin.

Green Beans (2.4-8.7mg Si/100gr.): Like green beans many beans and peas are eaten with the shell. Seventy percent of the Adventist diet is fruits and vegetables.

Parsnips (2.3mg Si/100gr.): Fresh, peeled and boiled.

Avocados without skin and stone (0.64mg Si/100gr.): Avocados are high in potassium (30% more than bananas) and are believed to reduced blood pressure and the risk of stroke.

Raw Fruit (0.1-2.5mg Si/100gr.): Seventy percent of the Adventist diet is fruits and vegetables.

The examples of local vegetables (e.g., red beets, potatoes, cucumbers, green beans, and parsnips) are commonly sold at farmer's markets in the U.S.A. and happen to contain relatively high levels of silica. The amount of silica in vegetables and fruit grown in Loma Linda may be higher than indicated in Table 23 because of local irrigation with silica rich ground water.

Adventists of Loma Linda, like the Donnelly family of Ireland, have adopted the habit of eating oatmeal porridge at least once a day. A major potential difference is oatmeal sold in the U.S.A. has been stripped of silica compared to the Irish oat porridge called sowans prepared by fermentation of the oats and husks.

Bama Yao Food

The people of Bama Yao eat three times more vegetables than fruit and prepare their vegetables by boiling, steaming, or stewing them, not by frying them. People eat only one to two meals a day and only consume 1,400 to 1,500 calories a day. Their diet is low in meat and fat[473]. The people of Bama eat primarily locally grown pumpkin, sweet potatoes, bamboo shoots, tomatoes, peppers, yellow corn, beans, and whole grains. The portion of the Bama Yao diet that is highest in OSA is the following:

Pumpkins (70-350mg Si/100gr.): In Bama Yao pumpkins including leaves and seedlings are stewed and eaten. Pumpkins grown in soil fertilized with calcium carbonate have only 70mg of silicon per 100 grams while pumpkins fertilized with calcium silicate have 350mg of silicon per 100 grams[474]. It is likely that irrigation with the OSA rich waters of Bama Yao results in OSA rich pumpkins.

Sweet Potatoes with skins (93mg Si/100gr.): Because of the low socioeconomic status of Bama Yao, it is likely that sweet potatoes are eaten unpeeled.

Bamboo Shoots (70-190mg Si/100gr.dry weight): The amount of silica in bamboo shoots varies with species[475]. The bioavailability of OSA from the silica in bamboo is only 1%[174].

Conclusion of Dietary Bioavailable Dissolved Silica

There have been many books written recently on the health benefits of the Mediterranean diet. Most of the ingredients used in this diet are summarized and ranked by their silicon content in Table 23. Like OSA rich drinking water there is magic in the Mediterranean diet that results in health and longevity. The dietary magic is water soluble OSA and water insoluble biosilifications of SiO_2, such as phytoliths. The OSA reverses aluminum accumulation in the body as shown in Table 1 and 2[64]. Both the biosilifications and OSA lowers aluminum absorption in the gut. Because of this magic, eating a diet of primarily vegetables and fruit has been found to lower the risk of three common fatal diseases:

- Cancer – Breast, Prostate, and Colorectal
- Dementia – Alzheimer's
- Cardiovascular Disease – Stroke and Heart Attack

Aluminum is a likely causal factor of all three of these diseases[1]. Lowering the risk of these three terminal diseases and thereby increasing longevity has been found to correlate with daily drinking silica water (see Chapter 3). We know that plants sequester OSA and other forms of silica for protection from aluminum (see Chapter 2). Therefore, by consuming plants, humans are ingesting the plant's stores of silica and using that silica for their own protection from aluminum.

Of the 10 most produced crops of the world 8 are silica accumulators and all 9 of the most produced crops in the U.S.A. are silica accumulators. In the U.S.A. production of these crops removes approximately 10 million tons of silicon that is equivalent to 34 million tons of OSA from the soil each year. Silica levels in these crops are declining because silica is not used as fertilizer. Silica supplementation to croplands does enhance both the yield and silica level of the edible portion of these crops. In the six longevity regions of the world crop irrigation with silica rich water provides a healthy OSA supplement to crops.

In all longevity regions, except Loma Linda, eating unpeeled potatoes or yams has either provided or currently provides the highest source of daily dietary silica second only to drinking silica rich water. In the U.S.A. most people peel potatoes prior to cooking and eating. For this reason, in the U.S.A. silica ingestion comes primarily from drinking water, but only in those communities with high levels of silica in their drinking water, such as Loma Linda. A secondary daily source of silica in Loma Linda is oat meal porridge.

Chapter 5 – Silica Water for Healing

"Fortunate is the person who is able to understand the causes of things" – Virgil 29 BC

Living in the Aluminum Age negatively impacts the health of everyone as we all accumulate aluminum just by eating and drinking. Where we accumulate aluminum in our bodies and how much aluminum we accumulate is subject to individual variation. This accounts for why aluminum accumulation impacts people's health in many different ways. This chapter describes healing from both aluminum accumulation and diseases and disorders in which aluminum is likely a causal factor. Facilitating excretion of aluminum by drinking OSA rich silica water allows us to heal from the toxic effects of aluminum and diseases and disorders caused by aluminum. It takes a resilient spirit to make a lifestyle choice of drinking OSA rich silica water, but as you will see in this chapter, OSA can heal aluminum damage and provide dividends in extended healthy individual longevity.

Aluminum Toxicity and Exposure

Before describing diseases and disorders in which aluminum is a causal factor we must talk about aluminum poisoning. Both acute and chronic aluminum poisoning is due to excessive exposure to aluminum. Because both aluminum and traumatic brain damage weakens the blood brain barrier (BBB), some humans are more vulnerable than others to aluminum's toxicity. This vulnerability has increased in the Aluminum Age because of increased exposure to aluminum containing products.

Acute Aluminum Poisoning

Aluminum ions kill neurons and for this reason it is accepted that aluminum is neurotoxic and neurodegenerative. The toxicity of aluminum ions in the cerebrospinal fluid (CSF) on the brain side of the blood brain barrier (BBB) is underscored by two patients who underwent routine brain surgery requiring bone cement. The cements used were of a new type that contained labile aluminum ions[209]. After the operations their CSF had 63-112mcg per liter of aluminum. The patients never regained consciousness and died 80-143 days after their operations[210].

In order to put this 63-112mcg per liter of aluminum in the CSF in some perspective, over half the alum treated surface drinking water in the U.S.A. contains aluminum at over 100mcg per liter (ppb) (see Table 20). So, aluminum in the CSF at concentrations found in most U.S.A. alum treated surface drinking waters would be considered fatally neurotoxic. There are two barriers preventing aluminum from being transferred from drinking water to the CSF: absorption from the gut to the blood and transfer across the BBB to the CSF.

In humans, acute aluminum poisoning has been studied in uremic patients who are on dialysis because of kidney failure. Acute aluminum poisoning is caused by high levels of aluminum in the dialysate, the co-ingestion of aluminum containing phosphate binders and citrate, or the rapid rise in blood serum aluminum following desferoxamine inoculation[211]. Desferoxamine is an FDA approved iron and aluminum chelator administered by inoculation for treatment of acute iron poisoning, but not for treatment of acute aluminum poisoning. In acute aluminum poisoning blood serum levels of aluminum are greater than 500mcg per liter where normal levels in the blood serum are only 1 to 3mcg per liter[212,213]. The onset of neurotoxicity is rapid and marked by confusion, muscle twitching, grand mal seizures, coma, and death.

Chronic Aluminum Exposure

Chronic aluminum exposure is very common in humans because aluminum is in drinking water, food, cookware, colored candy, pharmaceuticals, vaccines, and even inhaled air. Symptoms of chronic aluminum exposure are a gradual onset of neurobehavioral disorders and eventually death. These symptoms have been observed in both adults and children. Common neurological disorders that have been linked to chronic aluminum exposure are Alzheimer's disease, autism, multiple sclerosis, seizures, and Parkinson's diesease[1]. These neurological disorders and evidence that OSA rich silica water can be used to heal them will be discussed in this chapter.

Blood-Brain-Barrier's Role in Preventing Aluminum Toxicity

The blood-brain-barrier (BBB) saves us from certain death due to acute and chronic aluminum exposure. The BBB is made of cells (i.e., cerebrovascular endothelial cells) that are wedged tightly together to form a barrier that restricts the movement of ions, such as aluminum, between the blood and the brain. These cells are only the first layer of defense against aluminum entering the brain from the blood stream. The second layer of defense involves three types of cells on the brain side of the BBB called astrocytes, microglial cells, and pericytes. Primary factors causing increased BBB permeability to aluminum include:

- Aluminum[214-217]
- Traumatic Brain Injury (TBI)[218]

Aluminum oxide as nanoparticles, when exposed to human brain microvascular endothelial cells, decrease expression of the tight-junction proteins: F-actin and occludin[217]. This is not observed with nanoparticles of carbon[217]. Aluminum administered to juvenile rats also decreases expression of F-actin and occludin. F-actin is a protein for endothelial cell-to-cell adhesion and occludin is a plasma-membrane protein located at tight-junctions between endothelium cells[216]. Both of these molecules, whose expression is decreased by aluminum, are the "cement" that bonds the cerebrovascular endothelial cells together forming the first layer of BBB defense.

Once the first layer of defense is penetrated, aluminum can attack the astrocytes and microglial cells on the brain side of the BBB[219]. Aluminum ions cause inflammation in the brain by inducing both astrocytes and microglial cells to produce neurotoxic chemicals called reactive oxygen species (ROS) [219]. Aluminum is much more efficient than any other metal ion in inducing ROS production in human glial cells as tested *in vitro*[219]. This allows aluminum to penetrate the second layer of defense and enter the brain from the blood stream.

Two factors, aging and autism, and four diseases that are associated with increased BBB permeability are:

- Ageing[222]
- Autism - In autism aluminum is concentrated in microglial cells[65]
- Alzheimer's Disease[220]
- Vascular Disease – High Blood Pressure and Stroke[221]
- Parkinson's Disease[223,224]
- Lyme Disease[225]

Causal Inference and the Ladder of Causation

The study of causality has recently seen a major advance as described by Judea Pearl and Dana Mackenzie in their 2018 book entitled "The Book of Why" [453]. This advance is called causal inference and one of its accomplishments is construction of a mathematical query of causation expressed with a "Do" operator. For instance, longevity is increased in those people who "Do" drink OSA rich water and eat OSA rich vegetables. This can be expressed as the causal query: What is the increased survival rate (P) of 60-to-79-year-olds having sufficient longevity (L) to live to 90+ by ingesting OSA in water and vegetables. The mathematical form of this query is $P(L \mid do(OSA))$. The answer to this query depends on the longevity region. For instance, in Okinawa $P = 3.1\%$ for males and 5.8% for females (see Table 4).

In order to explain why silica water causes an increase in lifespan, a hypothesis is proposed and tested by the ladder of causation. The hypothesis proposed in this book is that since drinking silica water facilitates the excretion of aluminum from the body, aluminum accumulation in the body is a cause of shortened lifespan. This can be represented by the following causal diagram:

OSA → Lowers the Body's Accumulated Aluminum → Increases Longevity

Applying the three-rung ladder of causation this hypothesis can be tested:

- **First Rung – Association:** between **increasing aluminum exposure** and increasing rate of one or more terminal diseases. **Association:** epidemiology studies correlating aluminum in drinking water with increased incidence of one or more terminal diseases.
- **Second Rung – Intervention:** controlled experiments showing that drinking OSA rich water facilitates the excretion of accumulated aluminum (see Chapter 2). **Intervention:** controlled experiments to find if aluminum accumulation in the body is associated with terminal diseases. **Intervention:** experiments that test for aluminum modulating key biochemical pathways associated with terminal diseases.
- **Third Rung – Counterfactuals:** "It is a myth that aluminum causes terminal diseases" and "It is impossible that by drinking OSA rich water and eating OSA rich vegetables people can heal terminal diseases". **Understanding:** will negate these two statements.

From 2018, when this book was first published, to 2022 I continued using casual inference to climb 20 more rungs on the ladder of AD causation. This climb is summarized in my 2022 book "Finding a Cause and Potential Cures for Alzheimer's Disease". My current perspective from the 23rd rung is that aluminum is the primary cause of AD and drinking silica rich water is the best preventative and cure for AD.

Increasing Aluminum Exposure

Human exposure to aluminum has increased exponentially since the beginning of the Aluminum Age. The Aluminum Age began in 1888 when a low-cost process to purify aluminum from bauxite was developed by Karl Joseph Bayer. Since that time worldwide aluminum production has exponentially increased as well as the incidence of Alzheimer's and autism (see Figures 22 and 23). These neurological disorders are not ancient but instead have grown from only a few known cases to millions of cases over the last century of the Aluminum Age. These two disorders were discovered by psychiatrists with years of experience working with a single unique case that differed from all cases they had previously examined.

In 1888 Doctor Alois Alzheimer began working at a psychiatric hospital in Frankfort Germany. Thirteen years later, at age 35, Doctor Alzheimer started observing a patient named Auguste Deter. She had unique and new behavioral symptoms and had lost her short-term memory. After she died in 1906 her brain was autopsied by Dr. Alzheimer. Using special stains he found beta-amyloid (AB) plaques and neurofibrillary tangles (NFTs) and in his own words after translation:

"The case presented even in the clinic such a different picture, that it could not be categorized under known disease headings, and also anatomically it provided a result that departed from all previously known disease pathology"[226]

The prevalence of Alzheimer's disease has grown exponentially since 1906 and is simultaneously correlated with the growth of worldwide aluminum production as plotted in Figure 22.

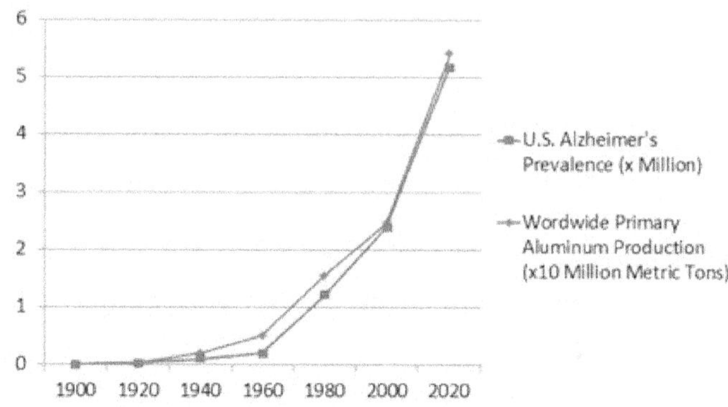

Figure 22 - Correlation of AD growth in the U.S and aluminum production worldwide[227-233]

In 1930 Doctor Leo Kanner began developing a child psychiatry service at John Hopkin's Hospital in Baltimore. Eight years later he started observing a child with a unique and new syndrome that he considered a modern disease. His belief is supported by the fact that it took him eight years working as a child psychiatrist to find his first case of autism and five more years to find 10 more cases. A child psychiatrist working in similar position today would find his first case of autism in a week, if not sooner. In 2016 it was estimated that 1 in 32 children born in the U.S.A. has autism. This corresponds to 110,000 autistic children born during 2016 in the U.S.A.

The prevalence of autism has grown exponentially since 1938 and is simultaneously correlated with the growth of worldwide aluminum production as plotted in Figure 23.

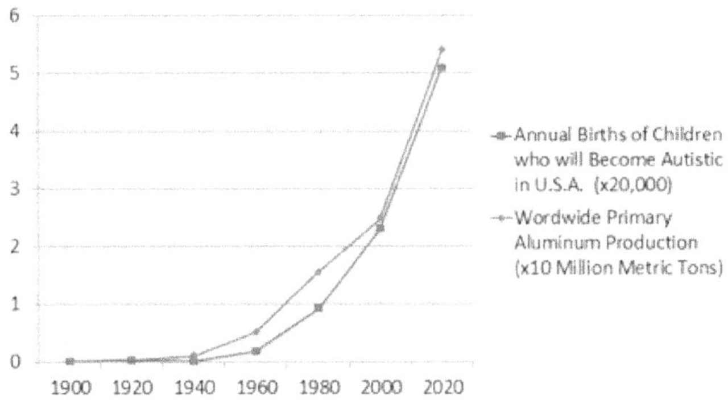

Figure 23 - Autism growth in the U.S plotted with aluminum production worldwide[1,227-229,234-237]

A relatively recent genetic mutation can't explain the approximate 80 years of exponential growth of both AD and autism. This is because during the last 200 years the average human generation time is 30 years with only three generations in 90 years[1]. What can explain the exponential growth of both AD and autism is an environmental factor whose production and chronic exposure to humans has exponentially increased since its introduction. Aluminum is a likely causal factor as it is currently used in drinking water treatment, food, pharmaceuticals, cookware, colored candy, vaccines, and inhaled air. Aluminum is also a likely causal factor because it is neurotoxic and causes neurodegeneration a common symptom of both AD and autism.

There are many modern mismatch diseases that are due to our evolved mechanisms for aluminum protection failing to protect us from an exponential increase in aluminum exposure[1]. In the following sub-sections of this chapter, mismatch diseases in which aluminum is a likely causal factor will be discussed. In all cases these mismatch diseases can be prevented and healed with supplemental OSA rich water and by eating OSA rich vegetables.

Alzheimer's Disease

My interest in silica water was inspired by a desire to help my mother slow or possibly reverse the progression of her Alzheimer's disease. I read Dr. Christopher Exley's work on daily silica water treatments improving cognition in some Alzheimer's patients and hoped this might work for my mom[73,78]. My research on Alzheimer's disease and ways to prevent it are summarized in my book "Prevent Alzheimer's, Autism, and Stroke with 7 Supplements, 7 Lifestyle Choices, and a Dissolved Mineral"[1]. The dissolved mineral mentioned in the title refers to the water-soluble silica called orthosilicic acid (OSA).

Alzheimer's disease is a terminal disease that slowly erases ones memory and identity. In the U.S.A. we are witnessing an exponentially growing epidemic of Alzheimer's (see Figure 22). Currently 700,000 people in the U.S.A. die every year from Alzheimer's making it the sixth leading cause of death. It is estimated that 1 out of 3 people in the U.S.A. over 80 have Alzheimer's.

But Alzheimer's is not an inevitable part of ageing. There are locations in the world, such as Japan and Okinawa, with a longer life expectancy than the U.S.A. and where there is much lower percentage of people dying from Alzheimer's than in the U.S.A. (see Table 24). These areas of the world have on average much higher levels of OSA in their drinking water than the U.S.A.

Table 24. Correlation Between Drinking Water OSA, Longevity & Alzheimer's Death Rate				
Location	ppm OSA In Tap Water	1970-2000 Male %Survival Rate[2]	1970-2000 Female % Survival Rate[2]	Alzheimer's Death Rate/100K
U.S.A.	11[3]	2.9	7.7	45.6[104]
Mainland Japan	26[12,13]	3.5	10.5	4.2[104]
Okinawa	40[14-16]	6.6	16.3	2.0[102]

In Table 24 both male and female survival rates are the percentage of people 60 to 79 who will make it to age 90 in each location. This table shows that both male and female survival rate to age 90 is higher in Mainland Japan (i.e., Honshu) and Okinawa than the U.S.A. The table also shows the Alzheimer's death rate in the U.S.A. compared with Mainland Japan and Okinawa is inversely correlated with average ppm OSA in drinking water. This OSA rich water is used for both drinking and crop irrigation.

The seven largest epidemiology studies looking at the link between aluminum in drinking water and the risk of Alzheimer's have found over 100ppb of aluminum in drinking water increases the risk of Alzheimer's[1]. In addition, several of these studies found a dose response relationship between the concentration of aluminum and the risk of Alzheimer's[238-246]. The good news is that one long-term study found that OSA greater than 18ppm in drinking water lowered the risk of Alzheimer's[246,247]. A second long-term study also confirmed that women over 75 drinking OSA rich water 19ppm to 57ppm were less likely to be diagnosed with Alzheimer's and had higher cognitive performance than women drinking water with less than 19ppm OSA[248].

Biomarkers for Alzheimer's

Three genes and an environmental factor (i.e., aluminum) have been linked as causal factors to Alzheimer's disease. There are three types and two sub-types of Alzheimer's disease (AD):

- **Sporadic AD** is the most common type (98-99% of AD patients) with two sub-types:
    - Those without E4 allele of APOE gene (44% of sporadic AD patients in U.S.A.)[249]
    - Those with one or more copies of E4 allele of the APOE gene (56% of sporadic AD patients in U.S.A. and 50% of early-onset AD patients)[249,250]
- **Familial AD** with presenilin 1 or presenilin 2 genes (1-2% of AD patients in U.S.A. and 35 to 75% of early-onset familial AD patients)[251]
- **Occupational AD** is the least common with at least one case of early-onset AD due to aluminum reported in the scientific literature[252]

Twenty percent of people in the U.S.A. have one or more copies of the E4 allele of the APOE gene. These people have a 50% greater than normal chance of having sporadic AD. This makes the APOE-E4 gene a potential causal factor of AD but not a reliable biomarker for AD (see "Aluminum and the Risk of AD in People with the APOE-E4 Gene" at the end of this chapter).

People with the presenilin genes are almost certain of having familial AD, making the presenilin genes biomarkers for AD.

In addition to these genetic biomarkers, there are three biomarkers common to all types of AD:

- Aluminum hotspots in the frontal and entorhinal cortex and hippocampus of the brain
- Neurofibrillary tangles (NFTs) of tau protein in the frontal cortex of the brain
- Beta-amyloid (AB) plaque in the frontal cortex of the brain

All of these biomarkers are visible microscopically in the autopsied brain with appropriate stains. The NFT's and AB plaque were discovered in 1906 by Doctor Alzheimer and the aluminum hotspots were first noted in 1973 by Crapper[253]. Recently there have been procedures developed for analyzing for these biomarkers in living patients (i.e., *in vivo*) by sampling cerebrospinal fluid or serum[254-256] or completely non-invasively by PET or MRI scans of the brain[257,258]. Retinal fluorescent lifetime and optical imaging of the eye has also been used to screen for some of these biomarkers[259-262].

Warning: *In vivo* detection of genetic and non-genetic biomarkers of Alzheimer's is in its infancy and suffers from high levels of false-positives and false-negatives. In addition, a percentage of the population can be resilient to the effects of some biomarkers. For example, 23.2% of a group of 966 people in two combined studies who had both a brain autopsy after death and comprehensive cognitive testing proximate to death were found to be resilient to beta-amyloid (AB) plaque in their brains. The 224 people found to be resilient had a significant amount of AB-plaque in their brains but no symptoms of Alzheimer's disease and were therefore without an Alzheimer's diagnosis at the time of death[263,264].

Aluminum as a Causal Factor of Alzheimer's

From aluminum analysis of the brains of those who had early or late onset AD and died of sporadic AD, familial AD, and occupational AD, it has been concluded that median levels of aluminum in excess of 2.0mcg per gram dry weight of brain across all four main lobes is both a common characteristic of AD and a contributor to its etiology[265]. There have been a total of 242 brains autopsied from people diagnosed with AD. In all cases these brains were found to have higher than normal levels of aluminum[252,265-267,486,487].

In 2005 aluminum levels in specific brain regions in three AD patients and three non-demented controls was measured[266]. The data in Table 25 shows regions of the brain where there were aluminum hotspots. In these regions aluminum is preferentially absorbed at higher levels in AD patients than non-demented controls[266].

Table 25. Aluminum in Brains from Humans with AD & Non-demented Controls[266]		
Regions of Brain Analyzed	**AD** **(Al mcg/g of brain tissue)**	**Controls** **(Al mcg/g brain tissue)**
Entorhinal Cortex	10.2 ± 9.0	1.5 ± 0.6
Hippocampus	4.9 ± 3.0	1.4 ± 0.6
Frontal Cortex (caudal)	6.8 ± 4.3	1.8 ± 0.6
Frontal Cortex (basal/ventral)	6.4 ± 2.9	2.5 ± 0.7

In 2011 Rusina et al. measured both aluminum and mercury in the hippocampus and associated visual cortex of 27 controls and 29 histologically-confirmed AD cases. There was a four-fold increase in aluminum levels in the hippocampus of the AD cases versus the controls. There was no difference in mercury levels between the AD cases and controls[267]. An amount as high as 8mcg/g of aluminum per gram dry weight of brain tissue has been found in the inferior parietal lobe of AD patients[268]. Hotspots in human brains with AD typically are in excess of 4mcg/g dry weight of brain tissue[268]. They contain a large number of NFTs or large pyramidal cells with high levels of aluminum. Hotspots are not found in non-demented age-matched controls[268].

It has been shown that a causal factor of all types of AD is environmental and not genetic[1]. Out of all environmental factors considered, only aluminum experimentally triggers all major histopathological events associated with Alzheimer's[269]. The "hotspots" in the brain where the highest levels of aluminum were found include the hippocampal complex, entorhinal cortex, and frontal cortex[266]. These areas of the brain are all important for memory. Impaired memory is the core clinical feature of AD. The entorhinal cortex had the highest overall aluminum levels, is amongst the earliest regions of the brain to develop NFTs, and is ultimately the most damaged region of the brain in AD[270-273].

Some brain atrophy in the hippocampal complex and the frontal cortex (i.e., 0.3-0.6%) is common with age in healthy adults[274]. In 2009 Fjell et al. studied brain atrophy in people 60-91 years old. The study included 142 healthy participants and 122 with AD. The four areas of the brain found to significantly atrophy during one year in AD patients were the same areas found to be hotspots for aluminum accumulation. Also, the rate of atrophy is much higher in AD brains than in healthy adult brains as shown in Table 26[275]. Of course, even healthy brains have accumulated some aluminum and that could account for the atrophy observed in the controls.

Table 26. Human Brain Atrophy with AD and Non-demented Controls During 1 Year[275]		
Regions of Brain Analyzed	**AD Longitudinal % Change**	**Controls Longitudinal % Change**
Entorhinal Cortex	-3.75	-0.55
Hippocampus	-2.42	-0.84
Frontal Cortex (caudal)	-1.60	-0.40
Frontal Cortex (ventral)	-1.06	-0.38

Note: these are the same brain regions found to be "hot spots" for aluminum accumulation[266]

There is ample evidence that aluminum is a causal factor of Alzheimer's, while there is evidence that AB-plaque and NFTs are merely symptoms of aluminum accumulation in the brain[1]. Currently billions of dollars are being invested in research to develop drugs for removal of AB plaque and NFTs from the human brain. Even if successful, these drugs will only provide palliative relief as they are only addressing symptoms and not a causal factor of Alzheimer's. I am not aware of any research dollars being currently spent on how to remove the causal factor - aluminum from the human brain. This is sadly ironic because on earth we have been blessed with low-cost silica to reverse aluminum accumulation.

Drinking OSA rich silica water daily has improved the cognition of many people suffering from AD in addition to my mother, now 96, who drank silica rich water daily for 5 years and still has enough memory to describe what she has done recently. This information comes from a facebook page my wife, Laurie Adamson, moderates: Alzheimer's: Late and Early Onset, APOE-4   https://www.facebook.com/groups/509038829797535 :

- *"I am the 3rd generation diagnosed with Alzheimer's. It runs very strong in my family. Possibly 5 generations as my Great, Great Grandmother and her daughter had memory problems before they called it Alzheimer's. The Fiji Water has been removing aluminum from my brain for almost 5 months and I can drive again and go shopping by myself again. Also doing memory block video puzzles. My scores are more than triple after starting detoxing from aluminum. I too thought it was over. But from first-hand experience I have learned you can improve a lot. No one should give up." Sept. 2020*

- *"I arrived in Kansas on September 13th and within 48 hours I had my mom on Fiji water. The changes include: She is much more communicative, involved in conversation, remembering events and telling stories, laughing, joking. She is no longer incontinent and knows when she has to go to the bathroom. Rarely does she have an accident whereas prior they could be changing her 7 to 10 times a day. ..... At almost exactly 2 months it was apparent that changes were taking place. My father even noticed and mentioned the changes. ...... She no longer just stares off like she isn't there. ..... Her short-term memory is poor but her whole personality has mostly returned as has her appetite ....I wish to give hope to others that while I don't believe Mom is "cured" she certainly has a much better quality of life than before I arrived to help and it has certainly made it ALOT easier for the caregiver." January 2021*

- *"I wanted to provide an update on my mom. She was diagnosed with moderate (stage4) Alzheimer disease back in November of 2019. Around November 2020 I started my mom drinking Fiji water (1 litre). Before starting the water, my mom's memory was getting bad. She couldn't remember her brother and sister's names, struggled cooking, had issues driving, wouldn't talk for more than 5 minutes on the phone. Since starting the Fiji water, she is able to understand when she says the wrong word and corrects herself, is cooking again, driving again, and she talks all the time on the phone with me! But most important, she is happy! I recently retested her and she is now at mild (stage 3). Thank you for all the information this group gives." April 2021*

- *"I'm 63 years old, not an Alzheimer patient (yet), but a little bit concerned about memory loss. For the last 6 months I have been drinking Volvic silica rich mineral water and I am really happy to feel that this 'brain fog' is disappearing, my confidence is back with no fear of driving, and I can again do calculations in my head". January 2022*

The Fly in the Ointment

Are the potential profits from future Alzheimer's drug sales or the current profit from aluminum sales preventing the evaluation of low cost and more natural solutions to Alzheimer's, such as adding supplemental silica to drinking water? Silica as a treatment does not fit the drug company's model of a successful drug (i.e., it is not a patentable pill or an inoculation that provides quick relief). Silica supplementation as a drinking water treatment needs to be both implemented by public health departments and embraced as an additive to domestic bottled water.

Obfuscation, paid for by the aluminum industry, has put aluminum research temporarily on hold. The aluminum industry has paid some scientists to publish articles on why aluminum does not cause Alzheimer's. Typically, these articles point out that people with kidney failure on hemodialysis have high levels of aluminum in their blood but don't have a high incidence of Alzheimer's disease. They fail to mention that people with kidney failure can't eliminate both OSA and aluminum by urination and have high levels of both of them in their blood as shown in Table 27[276,277].

With a working blood-brain-barrier, the OSA keeps the aluminum in the brain's cerebrospinal fluid at lower levels (i.e., 3-7mcg/liter) as shown in Table 27[276]. Approximately 4% of hemodialysis patients have a damaged blood-brain-barrier and die in a year or less due to aluminum quickly accumulating in the brain causing dementia (i.e., aluminum encephalopathy) in spite of high levels of silica. Since Alzheimer's disease takes 5 to 20 years before symptoms develop, hemodialysis patients with a damaged blood-brain-barrier die of aluminum encephalopathy long before they can develop Alzheimer's.

Table 27. Aluminum and Orthosilicic Acid in Serum and Cerebrospinal Fluid (CSF)		
Serum and CSF	**Aluminum** (mcg/Liter)	**Orthosilicic Acid** (mcg/Liter)
Normal Kidney Function		
Serum	<1	140 ± 40 (140 ± 14)
CSF	<1	235 ± 49
Hemodialysis Patients		
Serum	130 ± 8	4220 ± 630 (2190 ± 132)
CSF	5 ± 2	2580 ± 300

Data is from Van Landeghem[276] except for data in parenthesis from Roberts[277]

In 1998 a group under the leadership of J.D. Birchall found that high silica levels in the blood of hemodialysis patients lowered their aluminum levels[278]. They concluded:

> *"Further work needs to confirm a preventive role for silicon in the accumulation and subsequent toxicity of aluminum in dialysis patients."[278]*

For those hemodialysis patients with a working BBB, the silica and aluminum form HAS at the BBB preventing both Alzheimer's and high levels of aluminum in their brains[279].

Aluminum and the Risk of AD in People with the APOE-E4 Gene

The APOE-E4 gene increases the concentration of beta-amyloid peptide in the brain and has been linked to a higher risk of AD. The E4 allele of the APOE gene was introduced into the human population at least 1.5 million years ago[280]. The reproductive advantage of carrying the E4 allele was to promote human fertility in highly infectious environments in spite of its adverse effects on late onset diseases (i.e., an example of antagonistic pleiotropy)[281]. Because of this reproductive advantage the E4 allele frequency slowly increased during the last 1.5 million years with currently approximately 14% of the worldwide population carrying the E4 allele[280].

Because of improved hygiene and vaccines there is no longer a reproductive advantage to those that carry the E4 allele. In the absence of a reproductive advantage, the E4 allele frequency in the worldwide human population is not predicted to change (i.e., the Hardy-Weinberg principle).

Therefore, the recent exponential growth of AD is not due to an exponential increase in E4 allele frequency. Instead, the exponential growth of AD is due to a newly introduced environmental chemical that potentiates APOE-E4 making one of its protein products or their derivatives, such as oligomeric beta-amyloid peptide, more neurotoxic. This was proven to be the case by Denise Drago in 2008 when she tested a variety of metal ions (e.g., aluminum, iron, zinc, and copper) and found that only aluminum when bound to the oligomeric beta-amyloid peptide resulted in significantly increased neurotoxicity[282].

Aluminum is a causal factor of AD in people with and without the E4 allele of the APOE gene, but in those with this allele there is more oligomeric beta-amyloid for aluminum to toxify. For this reason, usually those with the APOE-E4 gene have a higher risk of AD than those without the E4 allele. **But what if there is an exception?** What if there is an undiscovered longevity region on earth where people with the APOE-E4 gene have the same risk of AD as those without the APOE-E4 gene? What if people in this undiscovered longevity region drink OSA rich water and eat an OSA rich diet that lowers their aluminum body-burden to the point where they are protected from the APOE-E4 gene?

The Exception – Ibadan, Nigeria an Undiscovered Longevity Region

The exception to APOE-E4 being a causal factor of AD is the Yoruba people of Ibadan, Nigeria who coincidentally have the same E4 allele frequency as people in the U.S.A. From 1992 to 2006 the APOE gene was genotyped in 2,245 elderly Nigerians living in the city of Ibadan who were also clinically diagnosed. Surprisingly, in contrast with other populations, the E4 allele in the Yoruba people was not significantly associated with AD or dementia[283].

The Yoruba people living in Ibadan are in general in better health than people living in the U.S.A. Age-matched annual incidence rates of both dementia and AD were found to be 2.4 and 2.2 times lower respectively, in a longitudinal study of a cohort of 2,459 elderly Yoruba people living in Ibadan versus a cohort of 2,147 elderly African-Americans living in Indianapolis, Indiana[284]. In addition, these elderly Yoruba people have lower incidence of vascular disease and vascular risk factors including hypertension than does the age matched cohort of elderly in the U.S.A.[283].

OSA in Ibadan's Drinking Water

Ibadan, Nigeria has a community water system that distributes water from the Eleyele reservoir. Tap water sampled at 11 sites across the distribution system indicated the water contained OSA at 22.4 to 25.6ppm[285]. This level of OSA in drinking water is approximately the same as average drinking water on mainland Japan (i.e., 26ppm) and more than twice the level of U.S.A. drinking water (i.e., 11ppm). This more than 2-fold increase of OSA in drinking water is associated with a more than a 10-fold lower rate of death due to AD in Japan versus the U.S.A. (see Table 9).

It is not surprising that both the Yoruba people of Ibadan and Japanese living on mainland Japan both have lower incidence rates of AD than people in the U.S.A., since OSA in drinking water lowers the body-burden of aluminum, a causative factor of AD. It is also not surprising that among the Yoruba people of Ibadan the E4 allele was not significantly associated with AD or dementia, since without a body-burden of aluminum there is no increase in neurotoxicity of oligomeric beta-amyloid. This is the peptide that occurs in higher-than-normal levels in those people with the APOE-E4 gene.

OSA in Ibadan's Food

Nigeria is the leading worldwide producer of cassava with annual production of 45 million metric tons[286]. Cassava, the most important dietary staple in Nigeria, is a tuber whose skin is very rich in OSA[286,287]. This makes cassava one of the richest vegetable dietary sources of silicon as OSA (i.e., approximately 270mg of silicon per 100 grams of cassava with skin that is equivalent to 920mg of OSA per 100 grams – see Table 23)[286,287].

The cassava root is toxic if not treated properly. Although cassava can be peeled with some difficulty, the tuber is usually cut into pieces with the skin on, dried, and fermented, in order to eliminate toxicity, and finally converted into three main foods by the Yoruba people[288].

Gari – granular cassava flour with a ferment flavor and a slightly sour taste is eaten in stews and soups and served with fried fish. Gari is also used as a snack when mixed with milk and sugar.

Fufu – cassava flour mixed into a paste with hot or cold water is ranked next to gari as an indigenous food of the Yoruba people.

Lafun – fibrous powdery form of cassava that is made into dough with boiling water.

The Yoruba people of Ibadan are a living example of how increased dietary OSA in their drinking water and food can lower the aluminum toxification of the oligomeric beta-amyloid peptide. This is the peptide that occurs in higher-than-normal levels in those people with the APOE-E4 gene. **By following the example of the Yoruba people of Ibadan and increasing dietary OSA by consuming OSA rich drinking water and OSA rich food, the risk of AD is significantly decreased in everyone either with or without the APOE-E4 gene.**

Silica Water Protects Amyloid Beta Regulation

Why are annual incidence rates of both dementia and AD 2.4 and 2.2 times lower respectively in Ibadan, Nigeria than in the U.S.A.? The answer is OSA in the drinking water and food of Ibadan's inhabitants protects amyloid beta (β-amyloid) regulation in their brains. Amyloid beta is a 36-43 amino acid peptide that is neurotoxic causing inflammation of neurons that can result in cellular death. Excess amyloid beta can also result in plaques in the brain that are a hallmark of Alzheimer's disease (AD). Due its neurotoxicity amyloid beta is normally regulated in the brain. Amyloid beta regulation involves not producing too much amyloid beta and quickly degrading the amyloid beta that is produced to non-toxic fragments. Aluminum interferes with both of these processes. Drinking OSA rich water and eating OSA rich vegetables facilitates aluminum excretion, thereby protecting amyloid beta regulation.

Amyloid beta is made enzymatically in the brain by a series of enzymes that cleave off chunks of amyloid precursor protein (APP). β-secretase 1 (BACE-1) is one of the enzymes involved in making amyloid beta. Aluminum epigenetically increases expression of β-secretase favoring the production of more amyloid beta[289,290].

Oligomers of amyloid beta (dimers, trimers, tetramers, etc.) are neurotoxic. Aluminum complexes of these amyloid beta oligomers are spherical droplets that are even more neurotoxic than amyloid beta oligomers[282]. Aluminum "freezes" the amyloid beta oligomer by inhibiting its further degradation to smaller fragments[291]. The rate-limiting step in the degradation of amyloid beta is catalyzed by the enzyme neprilysin. Aluminum epigenetically decreases expression of neprilysin that favors more amyloid beta in the brain[289,290].

Drinking OSA rich water and eating OSA rich vegetables decreases aluminum in the brain and restores amyloid beta regulation. In addition, OSA prevents amyloid beta oligomers from becoming more neurotoxic. Treatment for high levels of amyloid beta in the brain can also be done with aerobic exercise, and sleep. Aerobic exercise for 30 minutes increases the level of somatostatin in the brain that in turn decreases amyloid beta by increasing the activity of neprilysin[1]. Aerobic exercise also increases hippocampal volume[292]. In addition, sleep increases somatostatin expression and facilitates the purging of amyloid beta from the brain[1,293].

Conclusion of Alzheimer's Disease - Alzheimer's disease is the most common cause of dementia in the world. In Okinawa there is 52% less dementia than in Mainland Japan (i.e., Honshu) and 96% less dementia than in the U.S.A. (see Table 9). In Ikaria there is 25% less dementia than on mainland Greece. These longevity regions have less dementia due to higher levels of OSA in their drinking water and food. This OSA facilitates the elimination in urine and sweat of accumulated aluminum in the people's brains.

Aluminum is a neurotoxin that kills neurons in regions of the brain responsible for memory. In addition, aluminum causes neurodegeneration and brain atrophy in these same regions. Atrophy in these brain regions is seen in those suffering with Alzheimer's disease. There is ample evidence that aluminum is a causal factor of Alzheimer's[1]. In spite of this scientific evidence, the U.S. Alzheimer's Association, U.S. aluminum industry, and U.S. biopharmaceutical industry all actively deny the validity of this evidence establishing aluminum as a causal factor. In addition, they have failed to recognize the connection between OSA and aluminum detoxification as a preventative for Alzheimer's.

Removing aluminum from the human brain with daily OSA ingestion as a method of preventing and reversing Alzheimer's disease is based upon scientific evidence[73,78, 246-248]. The information in this book on how silica increases longevity also provides evidence that terminal diseases including Alzheimer's can be prevented and reversed with OSA in drinking water and food. As reported in this chapter there is anecdotal evidence that daily OSA ingestion reverses symptomology of Alzheimer's while improving the quality of elder life.

Atherosclerosis

Unlike many organs of the body in which silicon increases with age, such as kidney, brain, liver, spleen, and lung, silicon decreases with age in the plasma, aorta, and other arterial vessels[85,294,295]. The impact of less silicon in the circulatory system is development of atherosclerosis that is a general stiffening or hardening of the aorta and other arterial vessels resulting in higher blood pressure and a greater incidence of fatal coronary heart disease and stroke[296]. In the U.S.A. fatal coronary heart disease and stroke kill over three-quarters of a million people a year and are the first and fifth highest causes of death, respectively[297].

One of the first studies to reveal that dissolved silica in drinking water is an important factor in prevention of coronary heart disease was conducted by Klaus Schwarz. This longitudinal study was conducted between 1959 and 1974 and involved two groups of men: one group living in Eastern Finland and one group living in Western Finland[298]. In both groups smoking and obesity were approximately the same. The death rate from coronary heart disease was twice as high in the Eastern Finland group as in the Western Finland group. The only variable that could explain this large difference in coronary heart disease was the amount of silica in the drinking water as tested by Schwarz and shown in Table 28. The water samples were taken from private wells that had not undergone any changes for a number of years.

Table 28. OSA in Well Water Samples from Finish Longitudinal Study[298]		
Region	**Number of Wells Sampled**	**ppm OSA**
Eastern Finland	20	16.3 ± 0.9
Western Finland	20	26.3 ± 1.8

Coincidentally both mainland Japan and Western Finland have 26ppm of OSA on average in drinking water. While the U.S.A. has on average only 11ppm of OSA in drinking water (see Table 4). According to worldlifeexpectancy.com the death rate due to cardiovascular disease in men is 2.5 times higher in the U.S.A. than in mainland Japan. This is slightly higher than the factor of 2 differences in death rates due to cardiovascular disease in Eastern versus Western Finland. The 0.5% difference may be due to Eastern Finland having 5ppm more OSA in drinking water on average than the U.S.A.

Do high levels of aluminum in the blood cause coronary heart disease and stroke? This question was answered in an occupational health study of aluminum workers[299]. Forty workers exposed to aluminum while working in an aluminum factory were compared with 40 non-exposed subjects of comparable age who worked in administration at the same factory. The age range of the subjects was 18 to 62. The workers had been chronically exposed to aluminum dust levels of 0.33 to 3.4mg per cubic meter of air without any protective equipment. The study included a clinical examination of medical records as well as blood tests for aluminum. Aluminum blood levels of the exposed group were on average nearly 10 times higher than the control. The results of the clinical examination revealed a much higher frequency of both heart attacks and strokes in the exposed group. In fact, 5 of the 40 exposed workers had a stroke and 14 of the 40 had heart attacks. This compared with 2 cases of possible stroke with a symptom of a paralyzed limb (i.e., monoplegia) and 4 cases of heart attacks in the control group as shown in Table 29. Therefore, aluminum exposure is a likely causal factor of coronary heart disease and stroke.

Table 29. Comparing the Health of Aluminum (Al) Exposed to Non-Exposed Workers[299]				
Group	Al in Serum	Heart Attacks	Strokes	L-Carnitine
Aluminum	mcg/Liter	Number of Workers	Number of Workers	mcg/Liter
Exposed	24	15	5	7.0
Non-Exposed	2.6	4	Maybe 2*	15.9

'* 2 workers had a paralyzed limb (i.e. monoplegia) possibly due to strokes

Note that exposure to aluminum lowers L-carnitine in the serum by more than 50%[299]. L-carnitine acts as a chaperone that facilitates the transfer of large fatty acids into the mitochondria so they can be oxidized and metabolized for energy production. Aluminum lowers L-carnitine levels by inhibiting two enzymes involved in the biosynthesis of L-carnitine[300] and inhibiting the activation of an enzyme (i.e., MS) involved in the biosynthesis of a precursor of L-carnitine (i.e., methionine) from homocysteine[100,101]. Therefore, aluminum impairs the body's ability to use stored fatty acids as an energy source by lowering L-carnitine levels in the blood[299]. Low L-carnitine causes increased waist diameter and a larger body mass index (BMI) in adults[301,302]. A larger waist diameter is a negative biomarker for longevity in Nicoya (see Table 5). In the U.S.A. for each unit of BMI over 25 there is a 6% added risk of stroke for men[303]. In addition, aluminum increases the concentration of homocysteine[1] and homocysteine is a causal factor of atherosclerosis resulting in coronary heart disease and stroke[304-309].

Okinawans have low homocysteine levels in the blood as compared to westerners[99] (see Figure 10). This low homocysteine is in part due to the facilitation of aluminum excretion by OSA in their drinking water. Also, this low homocysteine may account for why Okinawans have less atherosclerotic narrowing and calcification and an 80% reduced risk for coronary heart disease compared to westerners. An autopsy of a 100-year-old Okinawan women in 2004 revealed normal age-associated changes in her heart. But remarkably her coronary vessels were free of atherosclerotic narrowing and calcification[96]. Autopsy reports on non-Okinawan centenarians show coronary vessel narrowing in 66% of centenarians and coronary calcification in 84% to 97% of centenarians[97,98].

Elderly Ikarians have more flexible aortas as compared to their peers on the Greek mainland[310]. This flexibility is due to less atherosclerosis that can lead to both stiffening of the aorta and an irregular heartbeat. Because of OSA rich drinking water, elderly Ikarians have good cardiovascular health, more flexible aortas, and 50% less heart disease than their peers on the Greek mainland[135].

The Nicoyan advantage does not occur in females and comes primarily from lower male cardiovascular mortality[146]. In Loma Linda drinking five or more glasses of OSA rich silica water a day was associated with a 54% less risk for men and a 41% less risk for women of a fatal coronary heart disease event compared with Adventists who drank only two glasses or less of OSA rich silica water a day[160].

Conclusion of Atherosclerosis - OSA in drinking water lowers the risk of coronary heart disease[298]. Aluminum exposure increases the risk of coronary heart disease and stroke[299]. Aluminum also increases homocysteine by inhibiting the production of methionine[100,101]. High levels of homocysteine in the blood are a causal factor of atherosclerosis resulting in coronary heart disease and stroke[304-309]. Based upon data from those living in longevity regions it is clear that high OSA levels in drinking water and food can facilitate the elimination of aluminum from the body, prevent atherosclerosis, and lower both homocysteine levels[99] and the risk of coronary heart disease and stroke by 40 to 80%[97,98,135,146,160]. Because fatal coronary heart disease and stroke are the first and fifth leading causes of death in the U.S.A., lowering their risk by drinking OSA rich water would increase both longevity and the quality of elder life in the U.S.A.

Autism

The links between autism and aluminum accumulation in the brain were described in my 2016 book "Prevent Alzheimer's, Autism, and Stroke"[1]. Autism is a modern mismatch disease in which our evolved mechanisms for aluminum protection are failing to protect us from an exponential increase in environmental aluminum exposure. For this reason, we are witnessing an epidemic of autism with the rate of autism in the population increasing exponentially since it was first discovered by Leo Kanner in 1938 (see Figure 23).

Unfortunately, aluminum absorption by the brain begins early in life. Aluminum is transferred from the maternal blood circulation to the fetal blood circulation via the placenta[311]. The brains of three fetuses, one full-term infant, and three premature infants from two to six months were analyzed for aluminum. These brains had a mean aluminum concentration of 1.2mcg per gram dry-weight of brain tissue with a standard deviation of 0.2mcg per gram[312]. Aluminum levels have been found to rise in the brains of fetuses during gestation and they rise the highest immediately after birth[313]. The blood-brain barrier that protects the brain is incompletely developed at birth and is even less mature in the human embryo.

Aluminum is introduced into the bodies of children by:

- Vaccinations with vaccines containing aluminum as an adjuvant
- Intestinal absorption from food, such as baby formula, colored candy, baking powder, drinking water, and a variety of pharmaceuticals, such as antacids
- Absorption through the skin from antiperspirants, astringents, cosmetics, and sunscreens

Aluminum salts injected into the body by vaccination slowly leach into the blood stream[1,451]. Approximately 50% of children with autism have increased intestinal permeability that is not seen in children without autism[129]. After a metal ion, such as aluminum, is ingested and absorbed by the intestine it becomes dissolved in the blood. Some of the metal is absorbed from the blood by the brain[451]. Also, an aluminum salt applied to the skin can become dissolved in the blood[446]. These routes of aluminum accumulation may be causal factors in childhood developmental regression of a subgroup of those with autism (approximately 25%) that lose skills as they age[314].

In 2012 an analysis was performed on hair from 44 children, age 3 to 9 years, diagnosed according to DSM-IV with ASD. It was discovered that the mean value for aluminum in the hair of autistic children (15.2mg/kg) was 90% higher than aluminum in the hair of non-autistic children (8.0mg/kg)[130]. This was the first analytical data linking high levels of accumulated aluminum to autism. In 2015 a second study demonstrated that aluminum levels in the hair of autistic children are higher than aluminum levels in non-autistic children. In this study the source of aluminum was traced to the use of aluminum cookware[315].

In 2017 an analysis was performed in Professor Christopher Exley's laboratory on the brains of 5 individuals with confirmed ASD, 4 males and 1 female. The mean and standard deviation (in parenthesis) of aluminum content across all five individuals for each lobe were 3.82(5.42), 2.30(2.00), 2.79(4.05) and 3.82(5.17) mcg per gram dry weight for the occipital, frontal, temporal and parietal lobes respectively. The highest amount of aluminum detected was 8.74 mcg per dry weight in the occipital lobe of a 15-year-old boy. These are some of the highest aluminum levels in the brain yet recorded and clearly link aluminum accumulation with the autistic brain[65].

In the brains of those with autism it has been found that the brain regions most impacted include the hippocampal complex and entorhinal cortex[316]. These areas of the autistic brain have smaller and less complex neuronal networks than normal[316]. This suggests a curtailment of normal neuron development and neuronal connectivity. These areas of the brain are also responsible for memory, learning, emotion, and behavior, disturbances of which comprise the core clinical features of autism[317]. Most importantly these are the same brain regions found to be hot spots for aluminum accumulation in the brain[266]. Glial cells that comprise part of the blood-brain-barrier were also found to be aluminum hotspots in the autistic brain[65].

In 2018 a biochemical classification of children has been found to have high (88%) reliability for diagnosing those with ASD[318]. This biochemical classification is based primarily on low levels of metabolites from two biochemical pathways serving as biomarkers of ASD:

- Folate dependent one-carbon metabolism (FOCM)
- Transulfuration (TS)

Both of these pathways are inhibited directly and indirectly by aluminum[1,100,101]. Therefore, low levels of these metabolites are biomarkers for both aluminum toxicity and ASD[455]. **The reliability of this biochemical classification of children is more supportive information that aluminum accumulation is a causative factor of autism.**

There has been no published study of silica water supplementation for elimination of some symptoms of autism. However, there is reason to believe that silica water may work to lower aluminum levels in autistic children and heal some symptoms of autism. The following is anecdotal information from Facebook and is provided by parents who gave their children OSA rich silica water for 3-8 months:

1. *"I have become fascinated with this subject and the unbelievable simplicity of drinking a silicon rich mineral water to remove aluminum from the body since discovering Prof Chris Exley's excellent work at the end of 2017. We have been using this on our 9 yr. old son who has an ASD (Autism Spectrum Disorder) diagnosis and we saw clear cognitive improvements with him after 3 months on Volvic water. There were improvements to his mood, his laughing. He was more happy and had more speech, asking significantly more questions (this is MASSIVE!), and more imaginative play. ... After 6 months on Volvic we switched to Fiji for the last two months and have seen dramatic improvements. He is so much calmer, better memory, understanding things more, eating more things and is generally eating more, will sit for dinner without requiring distractions, is laughing loads and showing emotions more, and is making progress which his teachers and tutors are also seeing. It's amazing to see! We have tried almost every protocol going since he was 3 and can confirm this is no placebo effect. This works, and is working for us and we hope more people try it with literally no down side. Amazing stuff!"* September 2018

2. *"My son is 21 and has autism. I started giving him Fiji water about 3 to 4 months ago. I didn't make him drink a certain amount or anything. He just drank it when he was thirsty, though he has always been a big water drinker. I didn't expect too much, but I can honestly say that I've noticed a difference! Mostly in the past month. I don't know how to explain it other than say he is more aware. Our conversations are getting to be more interactive. He initiated an 'I love you' for the first time in 21 years!!! Tonight, he said*

'Thank you Mom, you're the best!!'. This is not typical for my son. Not because he didn't feel that way, he just never expressed it verbally before. I'm not saying this to promise other parents that you will get the same results, but I'm very grateful for what we have experienced so far. I now buy a few cases of Fiji water a month as I truly believe it is helping". July 2018

The following anecdotal information is from Facebook and is provided by parents who saw improvement after giving their children silica rich water for just 6 to 8 weeks:

1. *"My daughter who is 12 has a moderate intellectual disability diagnosis as well as regressive autism level 2. She also had absence seizures and non-functional speech. Since starting Fiji water 6 weeks ago, 1/2 liter per day, she has been pointing to people and objects and commenting about them or asking questions - sharing an interest - the beginnings of conversation (which also had disappeared as she regressed). There has been a major change in her auditory processing as she now hears and responds to all speech. She is learning, retaining, and using information. **Absence seizures have stopped**, she is making eye contact, and receptive language has improved greatly where she now can follow 2-3 part instructions. I have seen changes in awareness, alertness, connection with others, conversation, and comprehension. It was like a light switched on. We have started and stopped the Fiji water especially initially. Improvements eased a bit upon stopping the Fiji protocol and picked up again upon restarting. I've done a lot for my daughter over the years but this has been by far the easiest intervention to apply with the most far reaching results across all areas for her". February 2018*

2. *"My 9 year old son has really struggled with reading. All of the sudden his reading skills have just taken off!! To the point his teacher wanted to talk to me after school! She said he has improved so much in the past 2 weeks she wanted me to know how proud she was of him! It is amazing he has only been on the silica water for about 6 weeks so I can't wait to see what the future holds." February 2018*

3. *My 6 year old son has been drinking about ½ liter a day of Fiji and I've seen big improvements in his behavior. Also much more affectionate. My dad commented that it's like he's grown up 2 years in the last couple months. August 2018*

4. *"I have been using Fiji water for my 3.5 year old son for the last 6 weeks. He is autistic and was preverbal. After starting Fiji water, there is a lot of improvement in his speech, understanding of language and memory. **He seems to have lost a bit of his chubbiness**, no other negatives so far." April 2018*

5. *I don't think my son would have improved this much or at all within this short timeframe (8 weeks). We get little improvements every now and then, but for this amount of improvement it would have taken at least 2 - 3 years-worth of hard work and still doubtful that he would have improved this much without the silica water. It is definitely the silica water that is all that is different with his diet. After 3 days of drinking it, very subtle things started happening and after one week, there was no way I was going to stop the water. I too was skeptical of whether this would work as you hear so many stories and things to try and not much seems to do anything, but silica water should be on prescription for ASD kids. September 2018*

6. *My 16 year old son has Aspergers, he has been using 800 to 1000ml of Ascilis for about 6 weeks with no side effects just positive changes. He was prior to starting socially awkward, antisocial, rather withdrawn and enjoying being alone and isolating himself in his room when he wasn't at school. Now he is a lot more communicative, quite enjoying online chats for hours with friends, chipping in family conversation, and being a lot more conversational and spontaneous. Initially I thought I was imagining things!! Even he says he feels different, clearer thinking and a bit more able to plan and remember what he's supposed to be doing, I have to say I am very impressed so far with the results. February 2019*

7. *I have been using Fiji water for my 7 year old who is higher functioning on the spectrum but used to not talk as much. Since the Fiji water, it's been 2 months, he has been so*

much more aware of surroundings; talkative and more curious about what is going on around him. Even in school his teachers have noticed a difference in speech. March 2017

8. *"We have been using **Silicade**. After 4 weeks my 7 year old autistic son showed no signs of improvement. But after 8 weeks on Silicade his hyperactivity had decreased allowing him to attend an entire church service. After 12 weeks he is continuing to improve, and I'm starting to worry that the special school section he's in may notice and kick him out!"*

Note: Silicade is homemade synthetic silica water with the same level of OSA as Fiji water. A recipe for Silicade is in Chapter 6.

The loss of weight (i.e., *"lost ... his chubbiness"*) seen in some children and adults after starting on silica water is likely due to a rise in L-carnitine in the blood. L-Carnitine acts as a chaperone that facilitates the transfer of stored fat as fatty acids (i.e., triglycerides) into the mitochondria so they can be oxidized and metabolized for energy production. Both the production of L-carnitine and the oxidation of fatty acids are suppressed by aluminum toxicity resulting in increased BMI, as described previously in this chapter[299-302,319].

Approximately one in five autistic children with intellectual disability and one in twelve autistic children without intellectual disability have epileptic seizures[320]. The anecdotal information that *"absence seizures have stopped"* has been followed by others who have also observed more control over seizures with silica water:

"My 6 year old son has epilepsy, acute confusionary migraines and autism. He has been drinking silica water and not only are his seizures and migraines much better controlled but he has gone from being more 2-3yr old level to almost right with his peers in most areas. Still he is academically delayed but actually learning now, he wasn't before." Feb. 2018

This anecdotal information is encouraging and gives us hope that OSA rich drinking water allows the brain to heal from aluminum accumulation and provides recovery from autism. Of course, supplemental silica water is only the first step. A diet high in OSA rich vegetables (see Chapter 4) and avoidance of aluminum ingestion (see Appendix II) are both suggested for ultimately stopping neurodegeneration by removing aluminum from autistic children's brains.

Autism Due to Vaccine Injury

Children's body-burden of aluminum from vaccinations exceeds that from dietary sources, such as baby formula[1,321,322]. By comparing ASD prevalence in 7 developed countries, it has been shown that both the number of aluminum-containing vaccinations and the scheduling of these vaccinations during the first 4 months of a child's life is strongly correlated with ASD prevalence. Those countries, such as Sweden, Iceland, and Finland, who schedule no aluminum containing vaccinations from birth to 3 months of age, have less than half the ASD prevalence when compared to the U.K. and the U.S.A. where babies are given aluminum containing vaccinations from birth to 2 months of age[323]. In addition, a positive correlation was found between autism prevalence and childhood vaccination uptake across the U.S.A. population[324].

It is estimated that aluminum accumulation due to childhood vaccination may be causal a factor in childhood developmental regression of a subgroup of those with autism (approximately 25%) that lose skills as they age[324]. Here is anecdotal information from Facebook on how silica water can turn around this regression due to aluminum in vaccines:

1. *"The reason I have got so interested in silica water is because of my grandbaby. He will be 2 in September. We believe he is vaccine injured because he completely stopped all talking and jabbering after his 1 year vaccines. He has gone backwards it seems. I first came across diatomaceous earth, then Fiji water, and now the local silica rich spring water. My daughter mixes his tea and juice with the silica water. I can say without a doubt it has changed him. He can now look you in the eyes, but before he would not make any eye contact. He has started jabbering more. My daughter texted me last night saying 'Mama it's like I have a completely different baby he is looking at me and jabbering and trying to say mama again'. So we are keeping this all up in hope's we get our little man back. But no more vaccines for us. She is still breastfeeding and I feel that has helped him a lot as well as keeping his immune system up."* August 2018

2. *My son, aged 9, has severe autism which he developed after vaccination. It took about 6 months from this final vaccination for my son to go from a loving normal developed boy to having full blown Autism. Our boy was in fact gone, replaced by a stranger. I saw Dr.*

Exley's report on silica water and though we might as well give it a go. ... I switched my son to Volvic Water about 4 weeks ago, within the first week we noticed slight improvements - good eye contact, sitting for longer, more verbal and is singing along to more adverts, some appropriate speech, and I actually got a cuddle and a kiss from him. ... My son is currently on Day 32 of drinking silica water (Acilis mainly, sometimes Volvic). He is currently very calm, reciting TV adverts, full of smiles, looking though his DVDs. I plan to carry on giving my son Acilis Silica Water. At the moment we have experienced no negatives of switching to silica water. I don't think my son would have improved this much or at all within this short timeframe (8 weeks). ... We get little improvements every now and then, but for this amount of improvement it would have taken at least 2 - 3 years-worth of hard work and still doubtful that he would have improved this much without the silica water. It is definitely the silica water that is all that is different with his diet. After 3 days of drinking it, very subtle things started happening and after one week, there was no way I was going to stop the water. I too was skeptical of whether this would work as you hear so many stories and things to try and not much seems to do anything, but silica water should be on prescription to ASD kids." Sept.2018

I recommend that the mother drink OSA silica water when breastfeeding. It has been shown that the mother gives almost all her silica to the baby during and immediately after pregnancy (see Figure 8)[85].

Look for aluminum or alum containing vaccines in Table 37 or for a more up-to-date table: https://www.cdc.gov/vaccines/pubs/pinkbook/downloads/appendices/b/excipient-table-2.pdf

Conclusion of Autism – Aluminum has been found in non-autistic brains of human fetuses, one full-term infant, and premature infants. These brains had a mean aluminum concentration of 1.2mcg per gram dry-weight of brain tissue with a standard deviation of 0.2mcg per gram[311,312] This demonstrates that aluminum from the mother's blood is transferred to the fetal blood circulation via the placenta and some of this aluminum normally accumulates in the fetuses' and infant's brains.

Two studies have found higher than normal aluminum levels in hair samples from autistic children. In addition, higher than normal aluminum levels (2.3 to 3.8 mcg per dry weight) have been found in the following regions of autistic brains: occipital, frontal, temporal and parietal lobes[65]. These regions of the brain known to be hot spots for aluminum accumulation[266] are the same areas of the brain that are responsible for memory, learning, emotion, and behavior, disturbances that comprise the core clinical features of autism[316,317]. These regions of the autistic brain have smaller and less complex neuronal networks than normal[316]. Therefore, since aluminum is a known neurotoxin, aluminum can be considered a causal factor of autism.

It is likely that aluminum accumulation due to childhood vaccination is a causal factor in childhood developmental regression of a subgroup of those with autism (approximately 25%) that lose skills as they age[314]. Aluminum is used as an adjuvant in many of the vaccines given to children (Table 37). Aluminum containing vaccines have been linked to an increased prevalence of autism and seizures. OSA rich silica water taken by mother and baby has been shown to heal autism and childhood developmental regression that is likely caused by aluminum in vaccines.

Anecdotal information suggests that a diet that includes silica rich drinking water allows the brain to heal from aluminum accumulation and provides healing from autism. It is likely this occurs due to OSA's ability to facilitate the elimination of aluminum from the brain.

Cancer

In the U.S.A. there is a 5.5-fold higher rate of breast cancer and a 7-fold higher rate of prostate cancer than found in the Okinawan longevity region (see Table 5). Non-vegetarian Adventists have higher risk of colorectal, breast, and prostate cancer than vegetarian Adventists (see Table 18). Could colorectal, breast, and prostate cancers be caused by aluminum accumulation and be prevented by facilitating aluminum excretion with supplemental OSA in drinking water and vegetable fiber in the diet?

Identical twin studies are an excellent way to access the heritable (i.e., genetic) versus environmental risk factors of cancer. In 2000 a twin study was reported on 44,788 pairs of twins in Sweden, Denmark, and Finland. Statistical modeling was used to estimate the relative importance of environmental and heritable factors in causing specific types of cancer[325]. The results of this study are in Table 30.

Table 30. Percent Risk of Environmental and Hereditable Factors Causing Cancer[325]		
Type of Cancer	% Risk Due to Environment	% Risk Due to Heredity
Colorectal	65%	35%
Breast	73%	27%
Prostate	58%	42%

In fact, except for certain types of rare familial cancers, such as adenomatous polyposis coli, the contribution of hereditary factors in the etiology of most cancers is thought to be minor. This reasoning is based upon the fact that it takes many generations for even a dominate gene to move through a population and for this reason genetics can't account for the dramatic growth in incidence rates of cancers, such as colorectal, breast, and prostate cancer, in certain age groups.

From the data in Table 30 we can see that environmental factors have the primary role in causing sporadic colorectal, breast, and prostate cancer. Since the rate of all three of these cancers is lower in some of the longevity regions, could aluminum play a role in their etiology allowing OSA to play a role in their prevention?

The etiology of colorectal, breast, and prostate cancer has been found to be linked to a gene that that is called *BRCA1* (note: "*BRCA1*" gene is in italics). When expressed, *BRCA1* produces *BRCA1 mRNA* that in turn produces a protein called BRCA1 (note: "BRCA1" protein is in regular font). This BRCA1 protein is responsible for error-free repair of double-strand breaks in DNA. When DNA is not repaired properly, there is an increased risk of cancer[109]. But **two conditions** can prevent the *BRCA1* gene from functioning correctly and preventing BRCA1 from acting as a tumor suppressor:

- **Hereditary** *BRCA1* mutation in germ line cells lowers BRCA1 production[107,111]
- **Environmental** epigenetic decrease in expression of the *BRCA1* lowers BRCA1 production[108,110]

Hereditary - Since germ cells when fully developed become sperm and ovum, the *BRCA1* mutations are inherited and carried for a person's life increasing their lifetime risk of some cancers[107]. For instance, *BRCA1* mutations are linked to 5-fold increased risk of colorectal cancers in women younger than 50 years of age[167].

Environmental - Epigenetics is the modulation of gene expression by environmental chemicals, such as aluminum, without causing mutations. Aluminum can be considered a causal factor of colorectal, breast and prostate cancer because it epigenetically inhibits the expression of the *BRCA1*gene preventing DNA repair by the BRCA1 protein[110].

As aluminum products have become more common the amount of accumulated aluminum in our bodies has been increasing[1]. With this increase in aluminum there has been an increase in colorectal, breast, and prostate cancer in some groups of people as described in the next three sections.

Colorectal Cancer

Colorectal cancer is the third leading cause of cancer death among adults younger than age 50, after breast and lung cancer in the U.S.A[326]. Colorectal cancer also has the second highest incidence rate among young adults after breast cancer in the U.S.A[326]. Have colorectal cancers been increasing among those under 50 in step with rising worldwide aluminum production? In general, the incidence of colorectal cancer is being kept in check by periodic colonoscopy and polypectomy in those over 50 years of age. But what about those under 50 who are in general are not checked for polyps with colonoscopy?

In 2017 these questions were answered by a group of epidemiologists at the American Cancer Society involved in Surveillance and Health Services Research. Rebecca L. Siegel led a study that used age-period-cohort modeling to understand colon and rectal cancer trends from 1973 to 2013 in different age groups in the U.S.A[327] Cohorts consisted of patients who were diagnosed with invasive colorectal cancer documented in the U.S. National Cancer Institute Surveillance, Epidemiology, and End Results (SEER) Program. The SEER program is the only source for historical population-based cancer incidence in the U.S.A.

What Siegel and her group found is alarming as incident rates of both colon and rectal cancer are dramatically increasing in those under 50. In fact, the incidence of rectal cancer in 20-to-29 year-olds is increasing at the rate of 2.4% a year. The data was grouped into cohorts based upon the decade during which people with colorectal cancers were born (i.e., birth cohorts). The number of people with these cancers was referenced as a ratio with the number of people with these cancers in a birth cohort born in 1949 and the data for 20-40-year-olds is plotted in Figure 24[327].

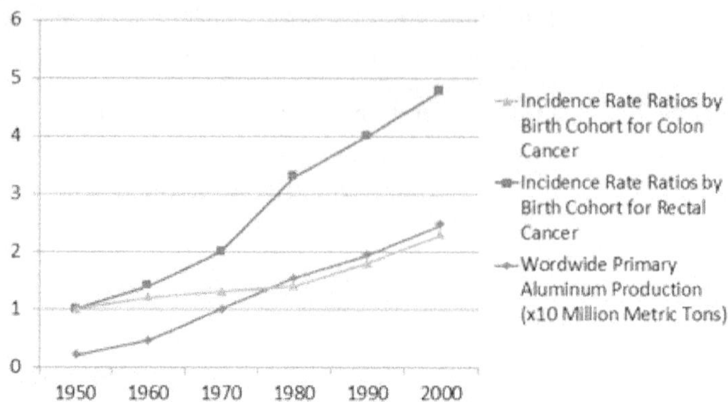

Figure 24 – Incident Rate Ratios for Colon and Rectal Cancer in the U.S.A. of 20 to 40 year olds. Based Upon Birth Date and Worldwide Aluminum Production[227-229,327]

By looking at birth cohorts Seigel disentangled the changes in medical practices, such as colonoscopies and polypectomy for those over 50, from factors that vary by generation. The data in Figure 24 clearly shows a correlation between the growth of aluminum production and rising rates of rectal and colon cancer in the U.S.A. particularly in those 20 to 40 years of age.

The risk of colorectal cancer is increased if either there is a germ-line mutation in the *BRCA1* gene[332] or the *BRCA1* tumor suppression gene's expression is reduced[107,108,110]. For instance, *BRCA1* mutations are linked to 5-fold increased risk of colorectal cancers in women younger than 50 years of age[167]. Aluminum epigenetically lowers expression of *BRCA1* resulting in reduced levels of BRCA1 preventing BRCA1 from suppressing colorectal cancer[110]

The lower rate of colon cancer in the Adventist population, as shown in Table 18, maybe due to both drinking more OSA rich silica water and eating more vegetables containing OSA[166]. Vegetables are good sources of OSA for facilitating excretion of aluminum in urine and perspiration preventing the development of colorectal cancer. An observational study revealed that in populations with low average intake of dietary vegetable fiber a doubling of fiber intake will reduce the risk of colorectal cancer by 40%[328]. This study involved over a half million people aged 25 to 70 years. The study followed almost 2 million people-years of data including 1,065 reported cases of colorectal cancer. The only studies of OSA in drinking water reducing the risk of colorectal cancer are those conducted on people living in longevity regions.

Breast Cancer

Breast cancer has the highest cancer incidence rate in women under 40 accounting for 30 to 40% of all cancer in females in the U.S.A.[329]. Breast cancer is the leading cause of cancer death among adults younger than age 50 in the U.S.A[326]. Young women with breast cancer tend to experience more aggressive disease and have lower survival rates than older women[330,331]. More aggressive breast cancer is called *localized* when it spreads to adjacent organs (e.g., lymph nodes, chest wall, etc.) and is called *distant* when it metastases to nonadjacent organs (e.g., bone, brain, lung, etc.).

Has breast cancer been increasing among those under 40 in step with rising worldwide aluminum production? This question was answered recently by using data from the U.S. National Cancer Institute Surveillance, Epidemiology, and End Results (SEER) database. Rebecca H. Johnson was lead author of a study that found the incidence of distant breast cancer in young women has increased from 1976 to 2009 as shown in Figure 25[331].

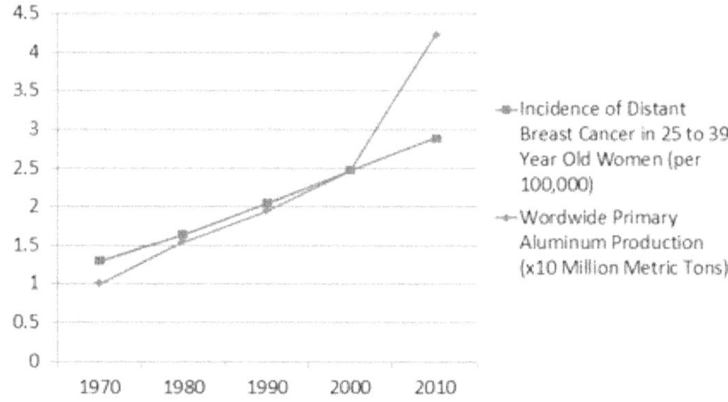

Figure 25 – Incidence Rate of Distant Breast Cancer in 25-39 Year Old Women in the U.S.A. and Worldwide Aluminum Production[227-229,331]

Although there appears to be a strong correlation between the rise in aluminum production and the rise in the incidence rate of distant breast cancer, this correlation does not extend to all ages of women and all types of breast cancer. In general, the incidence of breast cancer is not rising. One reason for this may be better early detection of breast cancer in older women than younger women with younger women being primarily diagnosed with more advanced disease. Another interpretation of this data is that aluminum accumulation is both a causative factor of cancer in breast tissue and cancer in nonadjacent "distant" organs. This interpretation requires that aluminum promotes both tumorigenesis and metastasis in mammary gland cells. **This has been shown to be the case as aluminum chloride at levels measured in human breast tissue promotes tumorigenesis and metastasis in mammary gland epithelial cells from mice[458].**

The risk of breast cancer is increased if either there is a germ-line mutation in the *BRCA1* gene[332] or the *BRCA1* tumor suppression gene's expression is reduced[107]. For instance, at age 50 the risk of breast cancer is increased by 28.5% for carriers of a mutated *BRCA1* gene versus those who are non-carriers[332]. More importantly aluminum epigenetically lowers expression of *BRCA1* resulting in reduced levels of BRCA1 preventing BRCA1 from suppressing breast cancer[110]. The aluminum salts used in antiperspirants, such as aluminum chloride and aluminum chlorohydrate, were shown to compromise DNA repair systems by reducing levels of *BRCA1 mRNA* in human breast epithelial cells[110]. *BRCA1 mRNA* is required for BRCA1 protein production.

The aluminum salts used in antiperspirants were also shown to cause double strand DNA breaks[110]. These breaks in the DNA also compromise DNA repair systems and increase the risk of breast cancer. **It is therefore not surprising that the use of aluminum containing underarm products, particularly starting under 30 years of age, is both significantly associated with increased risk of breast cancer and increased aluminum levels in breast tissue versus age-matched controls in a study of women with and without breast cancer[459].**

Prostate Cancer

The prostate is a gland in the male reproductive system and it is estimated that there will be approximately 165,000 new cases of prostate cancer in the U.S.A. during 2018[333]. About 99% of prostate cancer occurs in males over 50 years of age[334]. Prostate cancer accounts for 19% of male cancers and 9% of deaths in males due to cancer[333]. The incidence of prostate cancer is increasing worldwide. The incidence of prostate cancer increased in 32 of 40 countries examined during the decade 2000 to 2010[335].

The incidence of prostate cancer has been studied in Canada. Currently the age group in Canada with the highest rate of prostate cancer incidence is the 65-to-69-year-olds. When the incidence rate of prostate cancer in this age group is plotted against worldwide aluminum production there is a strong correlation with both having risen 4-fold between 1970 and 2010 (see Figure 26)[336].

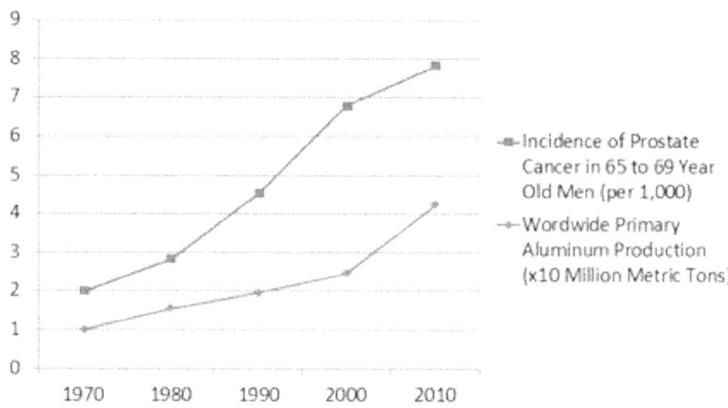

Figure 26 – Incidence Rate of Prostate Cancer in 65-69 Year Old Canadian Men and Worldwide Aluminum Production[227-229,336]

The risk of prostate cancer is increased if either there is a germ-line mutation in the *BRCA1* gene[332] or the *BRCA1* tumor suppression gene's expression is reduced[107]. For instance, at age 70 the risk of prostate cancer is increased 12% for carriers of a mutated *BRCA1* gene versus those who are non-carriers[332]. More importantly the risk of prostate cancer is significantly increased if the *BRCA1* tumor suppression gene's expression is reduced[107]. The *BRCA1* gene modulates proliferation, repair of DNA strand breaks, and expression of key cellular regulatory proteins in human prostate cancer cells. These activities are consistent with BRCA1 acting as a prostate cancer suppressor[111]. Aluminum epigenetically lowers expression of *BRCA1* preventing BRCA1 from suppressing prostate cancer[110].

Conclusion of Cancer - In the U.S.A. there is a 5.5-fold higher rate of breast cancer and a 7-fold higher rate of prostate cancer than those living in the Okinawan longevity region (see Table 5). Non-vegetarian Adventists in the U.S.A. have higher risk of colorectal, breast, and prostate cancer than vegetarian Adventists (see Table 18). A study of identical twins has shown that environmental factors account for over half the risk of having these cancers. Aluminum accumulation is likely an environmental causal factor in colorectal, breast, and prostate cancers. As shown in the longevity regions of Okinawa and Loma Linda these cancers can be prevented by facilitating aluminum excretion by drinking OSA rich silica water and eating a high OSA rich vegetable fiber diet.

Conception

Three meta-analyses have found that men from Western countries, such as the U.S.A., have declining male reproductive health[337-339]. One measure of reproductive health is sperm concentration in semen expressed as millions of sperm per cubic centimeter (a.k.a. cc). In 1998 Elisabeth Carlsen, et al., reviewed 61 studies (28 from the U.S.A.) on semen quality in men without a history of infertility[337]. The publications reviewed had studied 14,947 men between 1938 and 1991. Carlsen concluded there had been a genuine decline in semen quality over the previous 50-year period. Neils Jorgensen and Elisabeth Carlsen, et al., also published a paper in 2006 on semen quality in men from the Nordic-Baltic area of Europe[338]. Carlsen's data covering the 50-year period 1950 to 2000 is plotted in Figure 27. Carlson's conclusion has remained controversial until a more recent meta-analysis was published in 2017. This recent meta-analysis reviewed 185 studies on semen quality of 42,935 men and concluded from 1973 to 2011 the total sperm concentration in semen has declined 52.4% at a rate of 1.4% a year[339].

Sperm concentrations in semen below 40 million per cc have been shown to lower fertility[340]. The graph in Figure 27 shows an approximate three-fold increase from 1960 to 2000 in number of men with semen concentrations of less than 40 million sperm per cc of semen. This graph also shows the four-fold increase in world-wide aluminum production during this same time period.

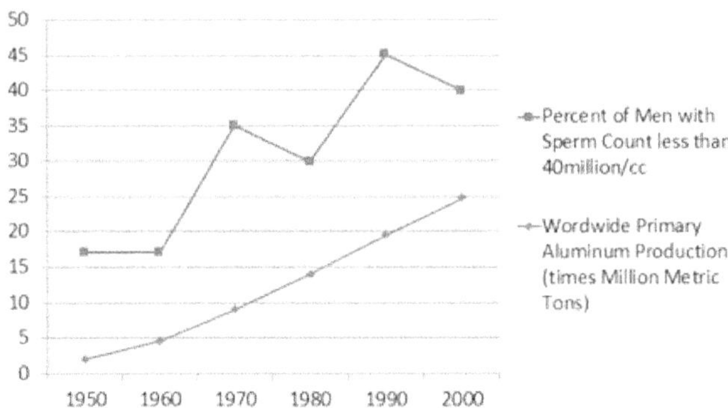

Figure 27 – Percent with Low Sperm Count and Worldwide Aluminum Production[227-229,337,339]

Spermatogenesis is the process by which sperm are produced by the testis. Aluminum has been found to inhibit spermatogenesis in rats and voles[341-343]. In the case of rats, the aluminum was administered orally at human dietary levels for just 60 days[341]. In 2014 aluminum was found in human semen at a mean concentration of 339mcg per liter with some patients having over 500mcg per liter. Patients with high sperm count had low levels of aluminum in their semen while patients with low sperm count were found to have higher levels of aluminum in their semen[344]. This was the first solid evidence that aluminum not only inhibits spermatogenesis in some mammals but also inhibits spermatogenesis in humans and is likely a causal factor in the decline of worldwide male fertility.

Sperm motility (i.e., mobility) is required for fertilization. In 2016 aluminum was found to inhibit human sperm motility[345]. There is evidence that aluminum lowers sperm motility by facilitating higher levels of reactive oxygen species (a.k.a. ROS) in the sperm[345].

Conclusion of Conception - The rise in worldwide production of aluminum is in synchrony with the rise in worldwide male infertility (see Figure 27). Aluminum has been found in human semen and higher concentrations are correlated with greater infertility[344]. Also, aluminum has been found to negatively impact spermatogenesis in other mammals (e.g., rats and voles)[341-343]. Finally, aluminum also lowers human sperm motility that is required for fertilization[345]. It is clear that aluminum is likely a causal factor of rising worldwide male infertility.

There have been no published studies of OSA rich water increasing male fertility by facilitating the excretion of aluminum. But hopefully these studies will be funded and published in the near future.

Multiple Sclerosis

Multiple sclerosis (MS) is a demyelinating disease in which demyelination of nerve cell axons occurs in the central nervous system (e.g., spinal cord and brain). Myelin sheaths on nerve cell axons electrically insulate the axons allowing them to very quickly transfer impulses. Oligodendrocytes are a type of glial cells that create myelin sheaths. Environmental chemicals that disrupt the biochemistry of oligodendrocytes will cause inflammatory demyelination lesions on axons, interference of axonal nerve conduction, and ultimately multiple sclerosis with a range of symptoms including physical, mental, and sometimes psychiatric problems. Cognitive impairment occurs in up to 65 percent of those with MS[346]. The specific symptoms of MS depend upon the location of the inflammatory lesions in the nervous system. MS is triggered by both environmental and genetic factors that increase the individual's risk of MS[347].

MS was first described in 1868 by Jean-Martin Charcot[348]. Approximately 2.3 million people worldwide were affected by MS in 2015 and 18,900 people died of MS worldwide in 2015 compared with 12,000 people in 1990[349]. MS is usually diagnosed between 20 to 50 years of age being most commonly diagnosed at age 30. Twelve twin pairs with identical genetics (i.e., monozygotic) were given a firm clinical diagnosis of MS in one or both twins. In 6 twin pairs only one twin had MS and in the other 6 twin pairs both twins had MS[350]. This suggests that the causes of MS include both environmental and genetic factors.

In 1980 the prevalence of MS was shown to have a strong dependence on the latitude at which people were living[351]. The number of deaths per year due to MS is a good indication of the prevalence of MS and this is shown globally in Figure 28[349]. Migration studies indicated that adult migrants generally retained the MS risk of their birthplace. However, it was found that those migrating under 15 years of age by moving either closer of further from the equator acquired the risk of their new residence[351]. A review in 2008 revealed that in the previous 30 years the MS incidence was both less dependent upon latitude and from 1955 to 2008 the female MS to male MS ratio had increased during this period from 1.4 to 2.3[352].

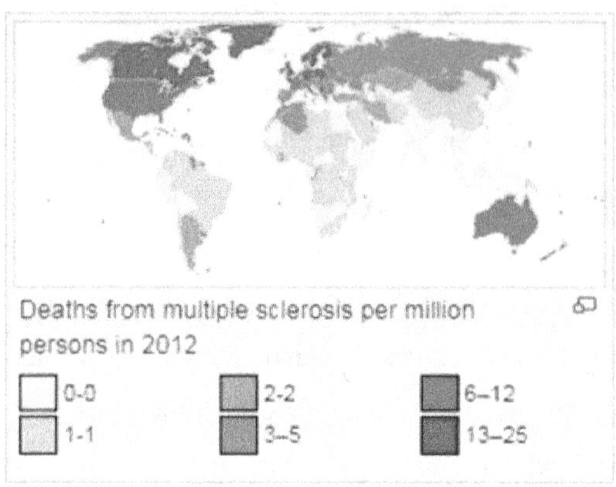

Figure 28 – Deaths from multiple sclerosis as a function of latitude in 2012[349]

The latitude dependence of MS is similar to that of autism in that both diseases are found at lower prevalence in the tropics[351,353]. Since the production of vitamin D3 in the body requires sunlight and there is more sunlight per day in the tropics, it has been theorized that vitamin D3 may play a role in preventing autism and possibly MS[354]. This role could be due to vitamin D's facilitation of aluminum elimination by the kidneys, even in children with chronic kidneys damage[355].

Although multiple sclerosis and autism have the same latitudinal dependence, the female to male ratio of those diagnosed with MS is the inverse of that observed in autism. It is known that young boys absorb more aluminum than young girls possibly accounting for why there are 4 times more boys than girls who are diagnosed with autism[128,129]. However, MS is a disease of women and men not young girls and boys. Women who are pregnant have almost no silica in their blood making them more likely to accumulate aluminum (see Figure 8) [85]. It is known that women who have unrecognized MS will start having MS symptoms during pregnancy or after delivery when they have almost no silica in their blood[356]. Also, up to 40% of women with relapsing-remitting MS will have a relapse after pregnancy[357]. This data agrees with the hypothesis that low silica in the blood during pregnancy results in more aluminum accumulation and MS symptoms in women.

The incidence rate of MS is rising at a rate faster than accounted for by either a genetic mutation moving through the population or improved testing for MS[358]. Three studies have been published that examined the temporal variation in MS incidence rates and the female to male MS ratio and the data is presented in Table 31 and Figure 29[359-361].

Table 31. MS Incidence Rates and Female to Male MS Ratios[359-361]					
Location	**Latitude**	**Years**	**MS Incidence (per 100,000)**	**Female to Male MS Ratio**	**Ref.**
S.E. Wales, U.K.	51°N	2006	7.30	4.3	359
		1983	2.65	1.8	
Newcastle, Australia	33°S	2001-2011	6.70	3.1	360
		1986-1996	2.45	2.0	
		1971-1981	2.14	-	
Tehran Province, Iran	36°N	2005-2006	5.68	3.1	361
		1989	0.68	-	

All three of these areas of the world have seen a dramatic increase in MS incidence in the last 20 to 30 years. Note that S.E. Wales is furthest from the equator and it does have both a slightly higher MS incidence rate and a higher female to male ratio than the other two locations.

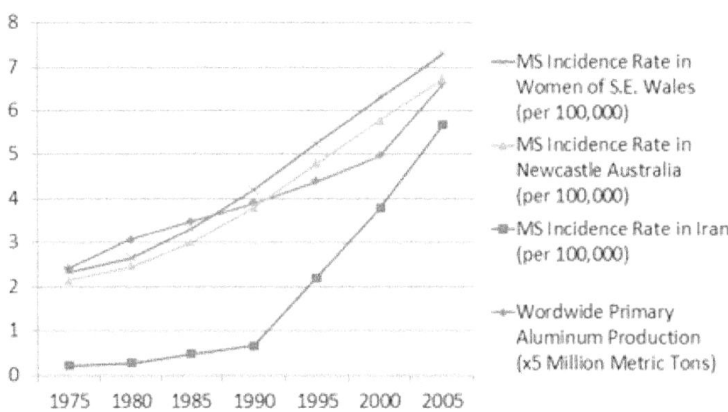

Figure 29 – MS Incidence Rates and Worldwide Aluminum Production[227-229,359-361]

In the thirty-year period from 1975 to 2005 the MS incidence rate of both S.E. Wales and Newcastle Australia increased three-fold[359,360]. During this same period worldwide aluminum production also increased three-fold. This rise in aluminum production has resulted in higher aluminum ingestion due to aluminum being added to drinking water, food, kitchen ware, drugs, vaccines, colored candy, and even inhaled air. These products increase both aluminum ingestion and aluminum accumulation in our bodies.

Multiple sclerosis is a demyelinating disease and myelin is made by cells called oligodendrocytes. Aluminum negatively impacts myelin production by promoting the peroxidation of myelin in oligodendrocytes[363,364]. Transferrin is a molecular iron transporter required by the body to move iron across the blood-brain-barrier. Aluminum can mimic iron due to similar size and ionic charge. Therefore, aluminum can be transported into oligodendrocytes by transferrin. When aluminum complexed with transferrin is incubated with oligodendrocytes there is a 3-to-4-fold increase in aluminum inside oligodendrocytes[362].

Table 32 - Metal Ion Induction of ROS in Human Glial Cells[219]	
Metal Sulfate	**Relative Induction of ROS**
Aluminum	10
Iron	6
Manganese	4.5
Zinc	4
Nickel	3.5
Lead	3.5
Gallium	3
Copper	3
Cadmium	3
Tin	2
Mercury	1.5
Magnesium	0
Sodium	0

Myelin is the preferential target of aluminum-mediated oxidative damage[363,364]. This oxidation occurs due to aluminum ions being transported by transferrin into glial cells, specifically oligodendrocytes[364]. Aluminum ions act as physiological stressors by stimulating brain cells to produce oxidizing chemicals (a.k.a. ROS) that cause inflammation in the brain[219,365,366]. Table 32 shows how much ROS is produced from a cell culture of human glial cells exposed to 50nM aqueous solutions of various common metal ions[219].

As shown in Table 32 aluminum tops the list of metal ion inducers of reactive oxygen species (ROS) in human glial cells, like oligodendrocytes. Aluminum at very low concentration (i.e., nanomolar) has also been shown to induce pro-inflammatory gene expression in human brain cells[366]. The accumulation of aluminum in oligodendrocytes causing inflammatory lesions is a likely causal factor of MS.

Chris Exley's group at Keele University has shown that people with MS have a higher-than-normal body burden of aluminum. They have also shown that OSA rich drinking water facilitates aluminum elimination in those with MS. The median daily aluminum excretion in the urine of people with relapsing-remitting and secondary progressive MS is 7.4 and 2.6 times higher, respectively, than people without MS[367]. The amount of aluminum excreted by those with relapsing–remitting MS was twice as high as people suffering aluminum intoxication. The median aluminum excretion in the urine of 14 out of 15 people with MS was found to 2.5-fold higher when drinking up to 1.5 liters of silica-rich water (35ppm OSA) per day with women excreting more aluminum than men[368]. Therefore, people with MS absorb and accumulate more aluminum than normal and silica water facilitates aluminum elimination in those with MS.

But do people with MS accumulate more aluminum in their brains than normal? This question was recently answered by Chris Exley's group at Keele University[369,488]. They analyzed brain tissue for aluminum from 14 donors with a diagnosis of MS and 12 donors without an MS diagnosis. They found that the aluminum content of brain tissue in those with MS was "universally high" with many tissues bearing concentrations in excess of 10mcg/gram dry weight and some exceeding 50mcg/gram dry weight[369]. Aluminum in the brains of those without MS was universally low with the majority of measurements below 1mcg/gram dry weight[488]. Aluminum specific staining showed aluminum both inside and outside of cells[369].

These results indicate that people with MS have a higher body-burden of aluminum than normal and some of that aluminum is in their brains at much higher-than-normal levels. Drinking silica-rich water facilitates the elimination of aluminum and possibly ultimately lowers the frequency of relapsing or slows the progression of MS.

There is limited anecdotal information available regarding OSA treatment for MS. But in 2014 a book was published titled the "The Wahls Protocol" written by Dr. Terry Wahls, M.D. [454]. Dr. Wahls was diagnosed with MS eventually requiring a wheelchair. But then miraculously she healed herself. She can now ride her bike as much as 18 miles in a day. This brings to my mind the biblical phrase: "Physician heal thyself" (Luke 4:23 King James Version). She changed her diet and a number of lifestyle choices that both increased OSA ingestion and decreased aluminum ingestion and accumulation for example:

- Consumed at least 6-9 cups of vegetables a day – Increases OSA ingestion (see Table 23)
- Consumed much more vegetables than fruit – Increases OSA ingestion (see Table 23)
- Added fermented vegetables to the diet – Increases OSA ingestion
- Reduced protein in the diet – Increases OSA ingestion due to substituting vegetables
- Switched to stainless steel and cast-iron cookware – Lowers aluminum ingestion
- Used sauna 4 times a week – Facilitates aluminum elimination that is enhanced with OSA
- Performed daily aerobic exercise – Increases hippocampal volume and produces more neuropeptide YY (a.k.a. PYY) that lowers aluminum absorption and accumulation[1].

MS Due to Vaccine Injury

The human papilloma vaccine (a.k.a. HPV, Gardasil) contains aluminum as an adjuvant and is given as a series of vaccinations to people aged 9 to 44. The HPV vaccine is primarily given to people at an age when they have the highest risk of MS.

In 2015 a Scandinavian study of 4 million girls and women age 10 to 44, of whom 800,000 were given the HPV vaccination, reported no statistically significant increased risk of MS[370]. Of the 4 million eligible for the study 5,553 individuals were excluded "because of prevalent multiple sclerosis" and 4,322 individuals were first diagnosed with MS during the study. However, of the 800,000 who received the HPV vaccination only 73 were diagnosed with MS during a 2-year period following HPV vaccination. However, 30-to-44-year-olds who were given the HPV vaccine were shown to have a slightly increased risk of MS diagnosis within 2 years of vaccination compared to those who did not receive the vaccine (40/100,000 versus 30/100,000).

The Scandinavian study did not evaluate the risk of a relapse of MS symptoms due to the HPV vaccine in those 5,553 people who were excluded "because of prevalent multiple sclerosis". These 5,553 girls and women are most likely to be both aluminum absorbers and negatively impacted by HPV vaccination. For instance, relapse of MS symptoms, for those diagnosed with relapsing-remitting MS, is likely triggered by either high levels of aluminum and/or low levels of silica in their blood. A study is needed to evaluate the risk of relapse after vaccination with an aluminum containing vaccine in those people diagnosed with relapsing-remitting MS. Currently the MS Trust in the U.K. recommends, if you are experiencing a relapse affecting your ability to carry out daily living activities, delay vaccination until your symptoms are resolved.

In 2018 in Miami, Florida two teens, one male and one female, who were 14 and 17 years of age experienced symptoms of MS within 1 to 2 weeks of vaccination with HPV vaccine[371]. They both were diagnosed with optic neuritis and had symptoms of **blurred vision** and in one case numbness and **weakness in the legs**. Oliogoclonal bands (i.e., bands of immunoglobulins) were found in their cerebrospinal fluid but not their blood serum indicating inflammation of the central nervous system that is indicative of MS. Both teens experienced a **relapse of symptoms** within 2 months of initial symptoms and were both diagnosed with relapsing–remitting MS[371].

MS is a disease with "obscure symptoms" [371]. Therefore, MS may fail to be correctly diagnosed in all cases. In the following anecdotal information from Facebook we may have an example of undiagnosed relapsing-remitting MS. Possibly due to both childhood vaccinations with aluminum containing vaccines and a diet of junk food and healed by drinking silica water and avoiding junk food:

*"My son has always been healthy, and I cannot remember a time where he has needed to go to the doctor in all of his 10 years. But at age 10 he went from healthy to wheelchair bound in the space of 6 months. First he had **blurred vision** and I noticed he was walking too close to walls and hedges, almost walking into them. Then he had chronic **weakness in his legs** and would fall over, unable to move his legs. He was tested and they found nothing wrong, believing it must be a mental problem. After all these tests he remained undiagnosed, untreated, and continued to deteriorate physically and mentally. I researched and followed Chris Exley's advice, giving my son Volvic silica water each*

*day. We noticed a difference within 3 days, he was out of the wheelchair within 10 days, and doing PE and gymnastics at school in 45 days. A **relapse of symptoms happened recently.** Unfortunately when my son strays off the healthy food and eats junk food over a certain amount of time, his symptoms reappear. Doctors don't want to admit that they failed and a daily bottle of silica water cured him. He has been on Volvic water since November 2016. This is something we will do for as long as we can. It is not a quick fix and needs to be a lifestyle change. Sorry to say it, the health system failed us, but Prof Exley's research saved our son. It sounds too simple to be true, but it worked unquestionably for us."* August 2018

Note that the symptoms in this anecdotal case (i.e., blurred vision, weakness in the legs, relapse of symptoms) are identical to those observed recently in Florida after HPV vaccination. These are likely examples of aluminum in vaccines and/or aluminum in junk food triggering MS or a relapse of MS symptoms. For more information on aluminum containing junk food to avoid and vaccines that contain aluminum see Appendix II and III.

Conclusion of Multiple Sclerosis - MS is a demyelinating disease that slows nerve impulses on nerve cell axons. The myelin that coats the outside of axons and associated glial cells (e.g., oligodendrocytes) that make myelin are targets for aluminum accumulation and toxicity[363-364]. In several areas of the world the incidence of MS is rising at the same rate as world-wide aluminum production[227-229, 359-361]. Aluminum ions are known to damage glial cells by stimulating the production of reactive oxygen species (ROS) [365]. ROS induced inflammation of glial cells results in inflammatory lesions that are characteristic of MS[347].

Compared with those without MS, people with relapsing-remitting MS have 7-fold more aluminum and people with secondary progressive MS have 2.6-fold more aluminum in their urine on average[367]. Also, people with MS have much higher than normal concentrations of accumulated aluminum in their brains[369,488]. Silica-rich drinking water has been shown to increase aluminum excretion in the urine by 2.5-fold in those with MS[368].

Further research is needed to find if a steady diet of silica-rich drinking water and/or OSA rich vegetables will lower the frequency of relapsing or the slow the progression of MS.

Osteoporosis – Low Bone Mass

Osteoporosis is the leading cause of morbidity and mortality in the elderly and has been called the "silent epidemic of the 21st century"[86]. Clinically osteoporosis increases the incidence of bone fractures of the femur, vertebrae, radius, and hip. These fractures in the elderly rapidly lead to a series of events that can result in death. These events include pain, disability, and loss of independence.

People living in the Okinawan longevity region have 20% fewer hip fractures than do mainland Japanese and about 40% fewer hip fractures than Americans[113]. The rate of bone mineral density (BMD) loss was compared between Okinawans and mainland Japanese. It was discovered that for women older than 40 and men older than 50, mainland Japanese lose more calcium from their bones than Okinawans[114]. OSA supplementation has been shown to improve BMD by both inhibiting bone mass loss and stimulating bone formation in humans[86-88] and rats[115-117]. Therefore, high bone density in older Okinawans is most likely due to high levels of OSA in their drinking water.

Bone Remodeling - Just like homes being remodeled, our bones are continuously being remodeled for optimal strength. Two teams of cells (i.e., osteoclasts and osteoblasts) are at work to adapt our bones keeping them strong enough to support the load we place on them without breaking:

- The demolition team – Osteoclasts remove calcium weakening bones & lowering BMD
- The rebuilding team – Osteoblasts add calcium strengthening bones & increasing BMD

The rebuilding team (i.e., osteoblasts) is stimulated by load bearing exercise and the sex hormones (i.e., estrogen and testosterone) and inhibited by aluminum accumulation. Women over 40 and men over 50 have declining sex hormone production and therefore have more bone demolition than rebuilding causing progressively lower BMD. In addition, as we get older we have progressively lower blood OSA levels and accumulate aluminum at a higher rate inhibiting bone rebuilding causing progressively lower BMD.

Aluminum Inhibits Bone Remodeling - Aluminum ions inhibit the deposition of calcium in bones. In humans with elevated aluminum due to dialysis it was observed that the aluminum causes softening of the bones (a.k.a. osteomalacia) by inhibiting mineralization and lowering both osteoclast and osteoblast numbers[372]. The uptake of calcium by the femur of calcium deficient rats was observed to be 43% less when the rats were fed 0.25% supplemental aluminum chloride versus rats fed no supplemental aluminum chloride[373]. Aluminum citrate was observed to inhibit chicken bone remodeling by slowing bone calcification by osteoblasts and increasing calcium loss from bones independent of osteoclasts[374]. *In vitro* mouse bone formation was slowed by aluminum ions inhibiting calcium uptake by the bone[375]. These results indicate that ionic aluminum exposure inhibits bone remodeling resulting in lower BMD and weaker bones.

OSA Removes Aluminum and Increases Bone Mineral Density - Increased dietary consumption of silicon is associated with increased BMD in animals, including humans, while silicon deficiency is associated with reduced BMD[87]. Studies have shown that supplemental OSA in drinking water stops the loss of BMD in the femur and tibia (i.e., upper and lower leg bones) by reducing bone demolition by osteoclasts (i.e., bone resorption)[115-117]. In addition, supplemental OSA stimulates osteoblast cells to rebuild bones[88]. Therefore, drinking silica rich mineral water will facilitate aluminum elimination, bone remodeling, increased BMD, and stronger bones.

Conclusion of Osteoporosis – Low Bone Mass - People living in the Okinawan longevity region have 40% less hip fractures than people in the U.S.A. This is most likely due to higher levels of OSA in the Okinawan drinking water. Increased dietary consumption of dietary OSA in drinking water and OSA rich vegetables have been found to stop the loss of bone mineral density (BMD). OSA facilitates the elimination of aluminum and thereby enhances bone remodeling, increasing bone rebuilding, slowing bone demolition, and making bones stronger.

Parkinson's Disease

The recent announcement that Alan Alda has been diagnosed with Parkinson's disease (PD) sparked my interest in writing this section. Recent papers on the rapidly rising incidence of PD and a link between PD and traumatic brain injury make it clear that we need to know more[376-378].

PD is a neurodegenerative disorder of the central nervous system that negatively impacts regions of the brain that control movement (i.e., motor system). The main motor symptoms are called "parkinsonism" and the most obvious are tremor, rigidity, and the impairment of the power of voluntary movement (a.k.a. akinesia). PD generally occurs in people over 70 but in 5-10% of cases does occur in people under 50, where it is called "young-onset PD". PD is the second most common neurodegenerative disorder after Alzheimer's and PD is also a terminal disease. The motor symptoms of the disease are due to dopaminergic cell death in the substantia nigra (SN) region of the midbrain leaving this region deficient in the neurotransmitter dopamine.

The cause of PD is believed to be a combination of environmental and genetic factors. Aluminum is an environmental factor whose prevalence is increasing at approximately the same rate as the rising prevalence of PD. For instance, worldwide death from PD increased 2.3-fold between 1990 and 2013 while worldwide aluminum production increased 2.8-fold in this same period[229,376]. In the U.S.A. the incidence rate of PD is also increasing at a rate comparable to that of worldwide aluminum production as graphed in Figure 30[377].

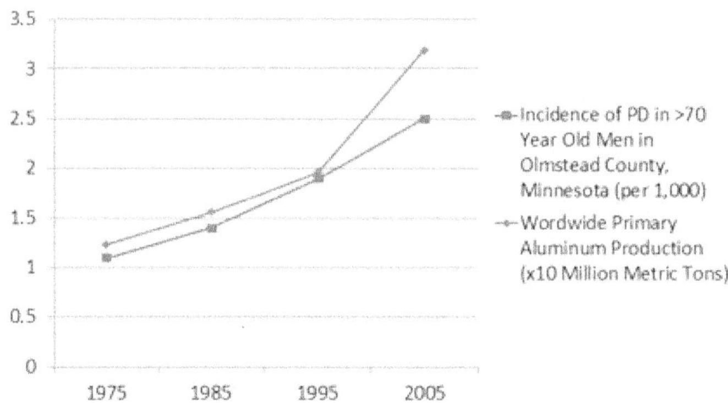

Figure 30 – PD Incidence Rates and Worldwide Aluminum Production[227,377]

Traumatic brain injury (a.k.a. TBI) has been found to significantly increase the risk of PD in later life. Records of 325,870 health care recipients of the U.S. Veterans Health Administration were studied. These records were age-matched 1:1 to a random sample of those with and without a diagnosis of mild to moderately-severe TBI. Those with mild TBI had 71% higher risk of PD than normal while those with moderate-severe TBI had 83% higher risk than normal of PD[378]. As explained earlier in this chapter both TBI and aluminum increase the permeability of the blood-brain-barrier opening the door to environmental chemicals, such as aluminum, entering the brain[214-218]. Aluminum and iron concentrations have been found to be higher in the SN region of the brain in people with PD as compared to people without PD[379-381].

Divalent Metal Ion Transporter (DMT1) is an iron transporter protein that transports essential iron to neurons in the SN region of the brain. Because iron and aluminum are approximately the same atomic size and can have the same electronic charge, DMT1 also transports aluminum that causes neurodegeneration in the SN region of the brain[382]. The amount of DMT1 being made (i.e., DMT1 genetic expression) is not governed by iron availability; but instead governed by a person's age and the brain location to which the iron is being transported[383]. For instance, DMT1 is increased for iron transport to the SN region as people age and is increased in the brains of Parkinson's patients[383,384]. The result is that as we age higher DMT1 expression in nigral dopaminergic neurons facilitates higher iron and aluminum levels in the SN region dependent only upon the availability of absorbed iron and aluminum[383,384].

Aluminum alters the metabolism of levodopa (a.k.a. L-DOPA) by increasing the ratio of dihydroxy-indole (DHI) to dihydoxy-indole carboxylate (DHICA) in SN regions that are slightly acidic (i.e., pH 5.5)[385]. A high ratio of DHI to DHICA inhibits the polymerization of a mixture of DHI and DHICA to neuromelanin (NM) [386]. Less NM means less protection from oxidative stress. Aluminum causes more oxidative stress (i.e., ROS) in the brain than any other common metal ion (see Table 32)[219]. Aluminum enhances both oxidative stress and dopaminergic neurodegeneration as has been observed in an experimental animal model of PD[387]. In the brains of patients with PD, oxidative stress leading to dopaminergic cell death is indicated by lower-than-normal levels of reduced glutathione (GSH) levels being found in the SN region[388].

Neuromelanin (NM) stores iron and can also store aluminum in neurons of the SN region. It is believed that iron and any aluminum stored in NM is less likely to cause oxidative stress and cell death in the SN region[389]. Normally NM slowly increases in concentration in neurons of the SN region from birth to age 90+[390]. However, patients with PD have only 50% of normal levels of NM, possibly due to aluminum causing a high DHI to DHCA ratio that inhibits the creation of NM[386,391]. This is a dangerous situation because people with a damaged-blood-brain-barrier[217,218] and all people over 77 years of age absorb and accumulate more aluminum than normal[194]. For this reason, accumulating aluminum that is unable to be stored by available NM, creates oxidative stress and dopamergic cell death in the SN region of PD patients[387]. Worse yet is when these cells die, a storm of NM stored iron and aluminum is released creating even more inflammation in the SN region of the brain[389].

Conclusion of Parkinson's Disease – Parkinson's disease (PD) is a neurodegenerative disorder of the substantia nigra (SN) region of the brain that is due to both environmental and genetic factors. The following evidence points to aluminum accumulation being a causal factor of PD:

- The incidence rate of PD is correlated with increasing worldwide aluminum production.
- Blood-brain-barrier damage due to TBI and/or aluminum increases the risk of both PD and aluminum accumulation
- Divalent Metal Ion Transporter (DMT1) genetic expression is increased resulting in the transport of too much aluminum and iron to the brain's SN region as people age
- Aluminum levels are higher in the SN region of the brain in people with PD as compared to people without PD
- Aluminum alters the metabolism of levodopa resulting in the inhibition of neuromelanin (NM) production and ultimately lowering NM levels by 50% in the SN region of PD patients allowing aluminum to cause oxidative damage to the SN region
- Lower than normal levels of GSH indicate oxidative damage to the SN region

Research on the etiology of PD has uncovered four causal factors:

- **Traumatic brain injury (TBI)** - Damages the blood-brain-barrier allowing environmental chemicals, such as aluminum, to accumulate in the brain
- **Divalent Metal Ion Transporter (DMT1) Expression** - is not governed by iron availability; but instead governed by a person's age and the brain location. DMT1 transports too much aluminum and iron to the brain's SN region in older people
- **Aluminum** – Damages the blood-brain barrier by decreasing expression of F-actin and occludin, generates ROS in human glial cells, alters metabolism of levodopa resulting in less neuromelanin, more oxidative damage and neurodegeneration in the SN region
- **Neuromelanin (NM)** – sequesters aluminum and iron protecting the brain from oxidative stress due to these metals. But people with PD have 50% less NM than normal

By drinking OSA and taking several drugs, PD can be both prevented and possibly healed:

- **Drink OSA rich water** – facilitates removal of aluminum preventing further damage to the blood brain barrier and oxidative stress, neuro-inflammation, and neurodegeneration in the SN region of the midbrain.
- **Non-aspirin and Nonsteroidal anti-inflammatory drugs (NSAIDs)** – NSAIDs decrease neuro-inflammation and reduce the incidence of PD by greater than 20% for long-term and regular users[393].
- **Levodopa** - L-DOPA combined with DOPA decarboxylase and COMT inhibitors is the recommended treatment for PD as they provide palliative relief from the symptoms of PD. Aluminum inhibits L-DOPA activation of homocysteine methylation by methionine synthase resulting in increased homocysteine in those with PD[100,381]. Therefore, OSA rich water is recommended in order to lower both aluminum accumulation and homocysteine.
- **Dopamine receptor agonists** – act directly on dopamine receptors mimicking dopamine and suppressing endogenous dopamine release. These agonists are recommended for younger patients with mild to moderate symptoms.

Preventing Alzheimer's Disease in Those with Down Syndrome

Children with Down syndrome have delayed growth, characteristic physical traits, and mild to moderate intellectual disability. Down syndrome (a.k.a. trisomy 21) is a genetic disorder involving the presence of all or part of a third copy of chromosome 21[394]. The extra chromosome occurs by chance with the parents of a Down child being genetically normal. The possibility of giving birth to a Down child is 0.1% in mothers 20 years old and 3% in mothers 45 years old. Currently there is no known environmental factor that changes these percentages.

Environmental factors do lead to earlier onset of AD in those with Down syndrome. There is a six-fold increased gastrointestinal absorption of aluminum in individuals with Down syndrome[395]. This is likely why 90% of those with Down syndrome over 30 years of age have similar neuropathology to Alzheimer's disease (AD) patients and at least 70% will develop dementia by age 55 to 60 years[395,396].

In general, as they age, people absorb and accumulate aluminum at different rates accounting for why some get AD earlier than others[77,397]. On average people under 77 years of age diagnosed with AD have a 64% greater gastrointestinal aluminum absorption rate than age-matched people without AD[398,399]. But on average all people over 77 years of age, with and without AD, have similar high rates of gastrointestinal aluminum absorption[400]. The major difference between AD patients with and without Down syndrome is an earlier onset of both gastrointestinal aluminum absorption and AD neuropathology in those with Down syndrome[401].

Conclusion of Preventing Alzheimer's in those with Down Syndrome - Aluminum does not cause Down syndrome but aluminum absorption is six-fold greater in individuals with Down syndrome than normal. This high level of aluminum absorption increases the risk of Alzheimer's in those with Downs resulting in 70% of those with Down syndrome developing dementia by age 55 to 60 years of age. In order to prevent Alzheimer's, it is recommended that those with Down syndrome take a daily OSA rich silica water supplement. In addition, a diet high in silica rich vegetables and grains is recommended.

Seizures

Epilepsy is a condition in which seizures occur on a repeated basis. Seizures occur in the brain when too many nerve cells "fire" too quickly creating what has been referred to as an "electrical storm". There are over 40 different types of seizures. Symptoms can either include convulsions, such as in tonic-clonic (a.k.a. grand mal) seizures, or no convulsions, such as in absence (a.k.a. petit mal) seizures. Other symptoms of seizures include: confusion, fainting, blackouts, blank staring, sudden and unexplained falls, episodes of blinking and chewing at inappropriate times.

The highest incidence rates of epilepsy have been reported in both the very young, particularly in the first few years of life, and the very old[402]. Currently the worldwide annual incidence rate of epilepsy is 68 per 100,000 people and in the U.S.A. the annual incidence rate is 35.5-38.6 per 100,000 people[403]. The Epilepsy Foundation estimates there are 326,000 children in the U.S.A. who have been diagnosed with epilepsy making it the 4th most prevalent neurological disease. Epilepsy not only lowers the quality of life of those who suffer its symptoms but also has a negative impact on their longevity. Two recent studies in Nova Scotia and the Netherlands have found that children with epilepsy are 5 to 9 times more likely to die than healthy children[404,405].

It is well known that aluminum causes seizures in monkeys. In 1954 it was reported that three months after aluminum hydroxide is injected in the brains of rhesus (*macaca mulatta*) monkeys, chronic epileptic seizures are observed in the monkeys that by EEG correlate with those in humans[406]. In 1978 chronic temporal lobe seizures were induced in 11 monkeys with bilateral implantation of aluminum hydroxide in their hippocampi[407]. The hippocampus is a known hotspot for aluminum accumulation in humans[266]. In 1982 chronic absence seizures (a.k.a. petit mal epilepsy) were induced in juvenile rhesus monkeys with bilateral implantation of aluminum hydroxide in their thalami[408]. Aluminum induced chronic epileptic seizures in monkeys have been shown to spontaneously continue for at least 7 years[409].

It is also well known that aluminum causes seizures in humans. Aluminum encephalopathy is a neurological condition due to aluminum accumulation in the brain usually occurring in humans undergoing regular dialysis treatment[410]. Epileptic seizures are observed in 57% of those diagnosed with aluminum encephalopathy[411]. Dialysis-associated seizures were seen in 7.2% of 180 children and adolescents on regular dialysis treatment[410]. Seizures have also been observed after 6 months of occupational exposure to aluminum and 36 to 42 days after the use of aluminum containing bone cement during brain surgery[413,414]. Serum aluminum concentration is normally less than 1mcg/L but in the cases of exposure to aluminum containing bone cement it was 4.4 to 4.3mcg/L[413,414]. High serum aluminum levels are a predisposing condition for epileptic seizures[476]. A person who drank water containing high levels of aluminum sulfate developed late-onset epilepsy and died of asphyxiation associated with an epileptic fit. Autopsy and analysis of their hippocampus revealed very high levels of aluminum (4.35 mcg/g dry weight)[477].

It has been reported that regular injections of an aluminum chelator (i.e., DFO a.k.a. desferoxamine) concomitantly lowered serum aluminum levels and abolished epileptic seizures[478]. Does supplemental OSA stop seizures by removing accumulated aluminum from the body? This question has been answered recently by a group of parents of children with seizures who had their children drink OSA rich silica water. The following anecdotal data from Facebook strongly suggests that routine OSA supplementation can in some cases stop seizures in children:

1. *"We started drinking Fiji water in January. It is now July and my child has been myoclonic jerk free since February. Honestly didn't think Fiji water was a factor so we stopped Fiji for two weeks just to see. Some jerks returned so we started it back up and so far none. We are sticking with Fiji". July 2018*

2. *"I have a similar story to yours. My 5 year old is still seizure free after starting on Fiji water. The last seizure was in November. I am not going to lie - sometimes I think it is not really the Fiji water? But seriously there is no other explanation!" July 2018*

3. *"We have been free from seizures for 11 months all from Fiji water." Sept. 2018*

4. *"We have been seizure free since March. Been using only Fiji since for all water intake." September 2018*

5. *"My son was on Fiji water for three weeks before we didn't see any more seizures. When we make ice tea or fresh lemonade, we only use Fiji water. Also, I dilute his juices with Fiji water. There have been times where he's gone 1-2 days without drinking Fiji water. He's been seizure free for one year now. I haven't even mentioned it to the doctor that it was after drinking Fiji water. I just don't want to hear how it is impossible that water can do such thing." September 2018*

6. *"My son is one month seizure free and 2 months since last seizure clusters. He has been on Fiji water for 2 months. I can't express how grateful I am for the Fiji water. It's amazing. My son has been having seizures for almost 10 years. For last 8 years, he had been having 10-20 seizures a month." September 2018*

7. *"We are going on 5 months of using Fiji water and have seen changes in frequency of my son's seizures from weekly to every 5 weeks. We are quite happy with the results as this has worked better than the different medicines we have tried." August 2018*

8. *"My daughter is 6 months seizure free today! She has never reached the six month mark before, so it's a pretty big deal. She has had no med changes but we switched her to Fiji water exclusively. Maybe it's coincidence, but maybe not!" – Oct. 2018*

9. *"My son has Dravet syndrome. We made a 100% switch to Fiji water. Things may have picked up a bit at first (not really sure since he was having so many every day). He went seizure free on day 9 and was for 30 days. After that the daily drops came back but not as frequent or as strong. Before Fiji he was falling on his face over 25 times every day. Since starting Fiji he hasn't hit the ground since. He went over a year on Fiji and never hit the ground." - Jan. 2019*

10. *"My granddaughter has stubborn infantile spasms as well and was also on ketosis when her mom put her on Fiji. The Fiji helped her go from hundreds a day to just a few. It was incredible!" - Dec. 2019*

11. *"We just got back from a trip to Mexico with our family. My son has epilepsy that is mostly resistant to meds. My son had a seizure the night before we left to Mexico. The resort we stayed at had strictly Fiji water! So we all were only drinking it. As I think back to the 12 day trip, he was swimming all day and definitely some later nights (seizure triggers being tired) but he did not have a seizure the whole time! Now was it a coincidence or was it the water!? I definitely won't be stopping the Fiji water anytime soon!" – Jan. 2020*

12. *"My daughter has autism and epilepsy and since starting her on Fiji water I have seen a big improvement with her. Not one seizure even when she had the flu just before Christmas, she has started talking, giving eye contact. I honestly can't believe the difference with her. I just switched my daughter to Fiji (she's always drank bottled water anyway). She has just under a liter a day and has been on it for 4 months." – Jan. 2020*

The results of an informal survey of 55 parents giving silica water to their children for controlling seizures revealed the following: 26 found at least 75% reduction, 12 found 25%-74% reduction, 3 found less than 25% reduction, and 14 found no reduction in seizures. Increased speech was observed by 43 of 55 parents after giving their children silica water.

Since OSA in Fiji water is known to only remove aluminum from the body, including the brain, these results give confirmation to the theory that in some cases accumulated aluminum in the body is a causal factor of seizures.

I do recommend starting OSA rich water slowly (i.e., one cup a day for adults and one-half cup for children) and then increasing to 3 to 4 cups a day, if there are no adverse side-effects (see Chapter 7 for side-effects). Both Fiji water and Silicade contain 124ppm of OSA and most children and adults do not have side-effects when drinking these silica waters.

Seizures Due to Vaccine Injury

Children get the largest amount of aluminum in their bodies from aluminum containing vaccines[1]. For instance, the DTaP vaccine, for diphtherias, tetanus, and acellular pertussis, contains the highest amount of aluminum (i.e., 375mcg) as aluminum hydroxide per dose of any vaccine given to children. Note that aluminum hydroxide causes seizures in monkeys[406-409]. DTaP vaccine is given four times at 2, 4, 6, and 72 months of age in the U.S.A. The warning given to parents regarding this vaccine is: "Talk with your doctor if your child has a seizure or collapsed after a dose of DTaP"[415]. Dravet syndrome is a refractory epileptic syndrome that is linked to inflammation following vaccination with vaccines containing aluminum adjuvants[479].

In order to prevent seizures after being given an aluminum containing vaccine it is recommended that you give your child OSA rich water for at least two months after a vaccination with an aluminum containing vaccine. The only caveat is there has been no study of vaccine efficacy as a function of OSA concentration in drinking water.

All ingredients in a vaccine, except the weakened or killed disease virus or bacteria that act as the antigen, are called excipients. The CDC maintains an online appendix of the "Pink Book" titled "Vaccine Excipient & Media Summary" with a table of "Excipients Included in U.S. Vaccines by Vaccine". Aluminum is an excipient and vaccines that contain aluminum are listed in Table 37. In order to keep current on vaccines that contain aluminum look for aluminum or alum containing vaccines in this table:

https://www.cdc.gov/vaccines/pubs/pinkbook/downloads/appendices/b/excipient-table-2.pdf

Seizures Due to Seizure Medications

Some seizure medications, such as ONFI (Clobazam suspension in solution), contain aluminum salts and may cause an increased frequency of seizures. Magnesium aluminum silicate, an inert ingredient in ONFI, is soluble in dilute hydrochloric acid as found in the human gut. Below pH 5.5 this compound releases aluminum ions in the human gut that are bioavailable.

"Clobazam solution contains magnesium aluminum silicate and when my son was on it, the longer he was on it the worse his seizures got, until we started Fiji." Feb. 2020

Stress and Inflammation Due to Reactive Oxygen Species (ROS)

Oxidative stress created in cells and tissues of the body by damaging reactive oxygen species (ROS) induces inflammation. Acute exposure to ROS is used by the body to control pathogens[416]. But chronic exposure to ROS due to environmental chemicals, such as aluminum, and the resulting chronic inflammation leads to variety of diseases including: atherosclerosis, chronic heart disease, stroke, cancer, rheumatoid arthritis, and cellular death[416]. ROS include superoxide (O_2^{*-}) and hydrogen peroxide that are partially reduced by-products of oxygen metabolism. These by-products are strongly oxidizing. Superoxide is produced by the electron transport chain in the mitochondria that provide cellular energy[416].

Aluminum ions make a bad situation worse by bonding to superoxide making aluminum superoxide[417] (AlO_2^*)$^{2+}$. Aluminum superoxide is a ROS that is claimed to be an even stronger oxidant than superoxide[418]. Therefore, aluminum creates more stress and inflammation due to ROS than another other metal (see Table 32)[219]. Aluminum also increases expression of two sets of genes that produce cell signaling molecules that promote inflammation and cell death:

- **Pro-inflammatory transcription factor: NF-KB -** initiates processes that are detrimental to brain cell structure and function. These processes result in inflammatory neurodegeneration of the central nervous system[419].
- **Pro-inflammatory cytokine: TNF-alpha** activates NF-KB and induces cell death particularly when exposed to excessive ROS generation and sustained activation of the enzyme caspase[416,420,421].

The following inflammatory diseases are associated with NF-KB activation by TNF-alpha and therefore facilitated by aluminum accumulation in the body: atherosclerosis, multiple sclerosis, rheumatoid arthritis, asthma, chronic obstructive pulmonary disease (COPD), inflammatory bowel disease (IBD), and ulcerative colitis[420].

Controlling stress and inflammation due to ROS in the body can result in longevity[421,422]. There are several ways of controlling stress and inflammation due to ROS and thereby increasing longevity:

- o **Drink OSA rich water** – facilitates removal of aluminum and prevents both the formation of aluminum superoxide and the expression of NF-KB and TNF-alpha
- o **Mitochondrial Superoxide Dismutase (SOD2)** – enzymatic conversion of superoxide to harmless oxygen and harmful hydrogen peroxide
- o **Catalase (CAT)** – enzymatic conversion of harmful hydrogen peroxide to harmless oxygen
- o **FOXO3A3 gene** – activation of the G allele of this gene by HSF1 leads to increased expression of SOD2, CAT, and GADD45A. The GADD45A repairs DNA damage done by ROS. HSF1 is a ROS stress relief factor that is increased in the presence of ROS[423]

Aluminum and superoxide make the perfect storm for increased ROS, leading to a number of diseases including terminal diseases, such as chronic heart disease (CHD), stroke, and cancer[420]. Removal of aluminum by drinking OSA rich water has the largest impact on ROS because, in addition to the production of aluminum superoxide, aluminum also inhibits the production of both SOD2 and CAT and increases expression of both NF-KB and TNF-alpha[417-419,421].

In 2008 a remarkable study was published showing that the G allele of the FOXO3A3 (rs2802292) is strongly associated with human longevity[422]. The study population was of Japanese ethnicity recruited from 9,877 Japanese-American men who were born from 1900 to 1919 and were mostly born in Hawaii and living on the island of Oahu in 1965. In most cases both parents of the study participants were born in Japan. In 1991 to 1993 blood samples and phenotypic data were archived at the commencement of the Honolulu Asia Aging Study that added 3,741 more male participants. In August 2007, 213 individuals who had lived to at least 95 years of age were grouped as "long-lived", wherein their mean age at death was 98.7. Also 402 individual who had died before 82 were grouped as "average-lived", wherein their mean age at death was 78.5.

This 2008 study showed that 62% of "long-lived" people had the TG or GG alleles of the FOXO3A3 genotype as compared with only 44% of the "average-lived" people. In addition, the "long-lived" people had 3.5 times less chronic heart disease, 2.26 times less stroke, and 1.47 times less cancer than the "average-lived" people. The study also demonstrated that those with the TG or GG alleles of the FOXO3A3 gene (rs2802292) were healthier than those with only the TT allele of this gene. But why is this specific gene allele associated with human longevity?

In 2018 the secret behind rs2802292 association with longevity was uncovered[423]. Those people lucky enough to have one or two copies of the G allele of the FOXO3A3 gene have a built-in ROS suppression system in their cells. When ROS is detected the ROS suppression system is tripped into action with a stress relief factor named HSF1. HSF1 and ROS activate expression of the G allele of the FOXO3A3 gene. This initiates a cascade of cellular ROS stress relief by producing the enzymes SOD2, CAT, and GADD45A. These enzymes detoxify ROS and repair any DNA that was broken by ROS.

Telomere Length as a Biomarker of Longevity

In the Nicoyan longevity region long telomeres were found to be a positive biomarker of longevity (see Table 15)[146,147]. Telomeres are pieces of DNA on the ends of chromosomes that protect the ends of chromosomes from sticking to each other. During cell division or mitochondrial biogenesis, a short piece of telomeres is lost every time DNA is replicated, ultimately leading to ends of DNA "fraying" and either cellular or mitochondrial death. Telomerase is an enzyme that repairs DNA by lengthening telomeres and thereby preventing DNA from having "frayed" ends. Telomerase increases both telomere length and the healthy longevity of cells and their mitochondria.

Homocysteine with ROS increase the rate of endothelial cell death by increasing the amount of telomere length lost every time DNA is replicated[424]. These effects of homocysteine are inhibited by the hydrogen peroxide scavenger catalase indicating that ROS is involved[424]. Aluminum not only promotes ROS formation it also increases homocysteine levels by inhibiting the methylation of homocysteine to methionine[100,101]. Metals that complex with desferoxamine (i.e., iron and aluminum) have been found to facilitate ROS damage to mitochondrial DNA including telomeres[425]. By drinking OSA rich water, Nicoyans remove aluminum from their cells and mitochondria thereby preventing mitochondrial DNA damage and death while keeping their telomeres long. By drinking OSA rich water Okinawans have low homocysteine that protects the endothelial cells that line their arteries from developing atherosclerosis (see Figure 10).

Conclusion of Stress and Inflammation Due to ROS - Chronic exposure to ROS due to environmental chemicals, such as aluminum, and the resulting chronic inflammation leads to variety of diseases including: atherosclerosis, chronic heart disease, stroke, cancer, rheumatoid arthritis, and cellular death[416]. Aluminum creates more stress and inflammation due to ROS than another other metal (see Table 32)[219]. Aluminum also increases expression of two sets of genes that produce cell signaling molecules that promote inflammation and cell death. The mechanism of FOXO3A3 gene acting as a ROS suppression system proves that decreasing oxidative stress due to ROS in the body increases longevity. **Therefore, since aluminum adds oxidative stress, it is not surprising that drinking OSA rich water to facilitate aluminum elimination from the body also increases longevity.**

Wrinkled Skin, Brittle Nails, and Hair Loss

If you are interested in living a healthy long life, I am sure you want to look your best along the way. The most visible effects of aging occur in the skin, hair, and nails. Restoring or maintaining a youthful appearance as you approach 100 years of life is a goal that can best be achieved on a diet that includes supplemental OSA. This is because silicon is an essential element required for metabolism of connective tissue that makes skin, hair, and nails[426].

Youthful skin appears soft and smooth. If you pinch youthful skin between your fingers and pull then release, the skin will snap back in place due to collagen. As we age our outer tissues lose their framework of structural proteins, such as collagen. Older skin sags and wrinkles as the collagen becomes weaker. OSA both activates enzymes that cross-link collage and is incorporated into structural proteins as a cross-linker[427,428]. This adds strength and elasticity to your body's structural proteins just as cross-linking with sulfur during vulcanization adds strength and elasticity to rubber. This strength and elasticity will allow skin to snap back in place preventing or removing wrinkles.

Silicon is also associated with the biosynthesis of glycosaminoglycans that help create the substance that fills the space between collagen and elastin[429]. Because of this the silicon in OSA is an essential component of healthy skin, hair, and nails.

Hair strands that have higher silicon content have greater brightness and a lower rate of falling out. Silicon is also an important component of healthy nails. In fact, soft and brittle nails can indicate a systemic silicon deficiency[429].

Chapter 6 – Supplemental Dissolved Silica

The primary reason for taking supplemental silica is to decrease the accumulated aluminum burden of your body's organs. This will lower the risk of diseases, such as Alzheimer's, atherosclerosis, stroke, cancer, multiple sclerosis, and seizures leading to greater longevity. In addition, supplemental silica may allow the brain to heal from aluminum accumulation and also provide healing from autism and improve male fertility. Orthosilicic acid (OSA) acts as a pH dependent selective chelator of aluminum. Unlike classical metal chelators, such as EDTA, that bind to a wide variety of metal ions, OSA binds only to aluminum hydroxide dimers at pH greater than 5.5 (see Chapter 2). For example, OSA does not bind to iron3+ that has the same ionic charge and approximately the same size as aluminum. Remarkable OSA supplementation even facilitates the removal of aluminum from bones that were once thought to be a stable sink for aluminum in the body.

OSA's remarkable ability to selectively facilitate the elimination of aluminum from the body has been proven in rats and humans. The following conclusions were reached with rats on a supplemental silica diet that involved oral administration of dissolved silica as OSA in water at concentrations of 200 and 400ppm for 5 weeks with and without supplemental aluminum as discussed in Chapter 2:

- In every tissue and organ tested, including brain, bone, liver, spleen, and kidneys, the prior accumulated aluminum is decreased by supplemental OSA[64].
- The reversal in aluminum accumulation is dose dependent averaging 58% with 200ppm of OSA and 79% with 400ppm of supplemental OSA after just 5 weeks[64].
- OSA at twice its saturation level in water (i.e., 400ppm) is more effective at lowering aluminum accumulation than at its 200ppm saturation level[64]. This implies that insoluble OSA, formed in supersaturated OSA, may bind to some of the aluminum in the gut preventing aluminum absorption[30].

Drinking OSA rich water at 50ppm to 160ppm, such as Fiji water and Silicade (both 146ppm), facilitates the elimination of aluminum in human urine[30,73,79] and perspiration[74]. Drinking OSA rich beer has also been found to facilitate the elimination of aluminum in human urine[79,80].

Drinking OSA rich water at concentrations over OSA's saturation level (i.e., 200ppm) without sufficient water for dilution can result in painful silica kidney stones. Likewise taking dissolvable OSA polymers or magnesium silicate without sufficient water for dilution can also result in painful kidney stones as discussed in Chapter 1. Therefore, the safest and most effective silica supplement is OSA rich silica water at a concentration of less than 200ppm.

See Appendix I for a list of international silica waters and a description of silica in beer.

The Good and Poor Silica Supplements

In order to lower the body's burden of accumulated aluminum the orally ingested silica supplement must be absorbed by the gut and travel in the blood to the organs. This is called silica bioavailability. The more bioavailable a silica supplement is the more effective it is at facilitating the elimination in urine and sweat of accumulated aluminum. **Therefore, a good silica supplement with high bioavailability is dissolved OSA rich silica water.** While a poor silica supplement has low bioavailability and remains in the gut to be excreted as feces and does not remove accumulated aluminum from the body's organs.

Some low bioavailability supplements are called "binders" and include plant fibers containing water insoluble biosilifications, diatomaceous earth, clays, activated carbon, zeolites, silica polymers, and colloidal suspensions of silica. Ingesting binders is not necessary because some of the vegetables, fruit, and grain we eat contain biosilifications that are very effective binders for aluminum in the gut (see Chapter 4). For instance 99.8% of the aluminum we ingest with food is not absorbed by the body and is instead bound to water insoluble biosilifications and excreted in feces. Some of the remaining 0.2% of aluminum can be prevented from being absorbed into the blood by drinking supplemental dissolved OSA during or after a meal[64]. Some binders, such as zeolites and clays, contain complexed aluminum that in the acidity of the human gut can become labile ionic aluminum that is absorbed. Table 33 compares the good and poor silica supplements by their bioavailability of OSA.

<table>
<tr><td colspan="5" align="center">Table 33. Silica Supplements[174,191]</td></tr>
<tr><td align="center">Supplement</td><td align="center">Dose/Day</td><td align="center">Silicon\Dose\Day</td><td align="center">Bioavailable OSA</td><td align="center">Cost/Day</td></tr>
<tr><td>Natural Waters[AK]</td><td>3 - 4 cups</td><td>30.5 – 40.7mg</td><td>44.8 – 60mg</td><td>$1.00 - $1.50</td></tr>
<tr><td>Silicade[BK]</td><td>3 - 4 cups</td><td>26.5 – 40.7mg</td><td>39 – 60mg</td><td>$0.04 -</td></tr>
<tr><td>Choline Stab OSA[DK]</td><td>10 drops</td><td>10mg</td><td>5.8mg</td><td>$0.42</td></tr>
<tr><td>Choline Stab OSA[EK]</td><td>2 veg caps</td><td>10mg</td><td>5.8mg</td><td>$0.83</td></tr>
<tr><td>Colloidal Silica[F]</td><td>30 drops</td><td>175mg</td><td>0.51mg</td><td>$0.60</td></tr>
<tr><td>Colloidal Silica[G]</td><td>10cc</td><td>163mg</td><td>1.36mg</td><td>$0.59</td></tr>
<tr><td>Bamboo[H]</td><td>1cap(300mg)</td><td>99mg</td><td>0.99mg</td><td>$0.10</td></tr>
<tr><td>Horsetail[I]</td><td>1cap(500mg)</td><td>16.5mg</td><td>0.37mg</td><td>$0.04</td></tr>
<tr><td>Diatomaceous</td><td>625mg</td><td><2.9mg</td><td>0.24mg</td><td>$0.01</td></tr>
</table>

A. Fiji – natural water; B. Silicade – synthetic silica water; C. Excluding cost of tap water; D. Biosil Choline Stab. OSA; E. Biosil Veg Caps;   F. Eidon – Ionic Minerals Silica Concentrate; G. Saguna – Silicolgel Colloidal OSA; H. Swanson; I. Swanson; J. Swanson
K. Samples acidified to pH3.2 for 4 hours all other samples for 24 hours prior to testing for OSA

The only recommended supplements are three to four cups a day of OSA rich silica water (e.g., natural such as Fiji or synthetic such as Silicade) as a daily supplement[1]. The half-life of absorbed OSA in the blood is approximately 3 hours[79]. Therefore, drinking a cup of OSA rich silica water every 3 to 4 hours during the day is the optimal strategy for aluminum elimination. Most people do not have side-effects when drinking 3 to 4 cups of OSA rich silica water over a period of 9 to 12 hours during the day (see Chapter 7 for side-effects). However, if you do have suspected side-effects, cut back to 1 cup a day and slowly increase to 3 to 4 cups a day.

Choline stabilized OSA, sold as Biosil, is a combination of 200mg of choline with 10mg of silicon as silica. Only 17% of the silica in Biosil is bioavailable as OSA compared with 43% bioavailability with natural waters and Silicade. Also, there is a 70% greater risk of lethal prostate cancer with high (500mg/day) choline diets[430]. Therefore, The European Food Safety Authority recommends that liquid choline stabilized OSA be taken at a maximum dose of 10 drops equivalent to 10 mg. of silicon complexed with 200mg of choline per day[431,432]. Also, since the use of Biosil in children has not been studied, the Biosil Corporation does not recommend it to be taken by children under age seven.

Natural OSA Rich Silica Water Supplements

Good silica supplements are high in dissolved OSA and include natural OSA rich silica waters and beers. The commercially available natural OSA rich silica waters that I have tested are indicated with a "*" and there is a more comprehensive list of silica waters in Appendix I:

- Starkey Spring Water from Idaho is available from Whole Foods (94ppm OSA*)
- Fiji water from Fiji is available in the U.S.A. (146ppm OSA*)
- Langkawi Pure from Malaysia is available in Asia and U.S.A. (133ppm OSA*)
- Volvic water from France is available in the U.S.A. and Europe (51 ppm OSA*)
- Gerolsteiner from Germany is available in Europe (64ppm OSA*)
- Acilis water from Malaysia is available in Europe (88ppm OSA)

OSA is present in beer, non-alcoholic beer, wine, and some sprits. The grain used for brewing beer adds dissolved silica during preparation. The mean OSA level of 76 different beers was found to be 65.3ppm OSA[191]. Some of these beers have high levels of OSA, such as the non-alcoholic beer Clausthaler Premium with 118ppm of OSA[79]. Appendix I has a list of the amounts of OSA in different types of beer.

Synthetic OSA Rich Silica Water Supplement

In 2009 synthetic silica water, like Silicade, but containing only 73ppm of OSA was made and tested for its bioavailability in healthy human volunteers 19-40 years of age (16 males and 16 females)[79]. Urinary silicon was used as a surrogate maker of bioavailable silicon[17,192]. The percentage of silicon excreted in the urine over a 6-hour period was 43.1% $\pm$ 3.6% making it one of the best sources of supplemental silica available. Serum silicon was also measured during this 6-hour period and was found to start at 120 mcg/liter, peak at 670 mcg/liter after 2 hours, and then decline slowly to 200 mcg/liter after 6 hours[79]. In 2000 synthetic silica water was shown to enhance 26-aluminum radioisotope excretion by 75% in several volunteers[30]. This demonstrates that synthetic silica is absorbed in the gut, dissolved in the blood, collected by the kidneys, excreted in the urine, and enhances urinary aluminum excretion.

This synthetic silica water was made from concentrated liquid alkaline sodium silicate that was purchased from the Aldrich Chemical Company (7 mol Si/liter containing 10.5% as Na_2O and 27% SiO_2 with a SiO_2 to Na_2O ratio of 3.22). The procedure involved diluting the basic sodium silicate in water and then acidifying with hydrochloric acid to pH 7.0 – 7.2. The final solutions contained 73ppm OSA (21.4 mg Si) as measured by inductively coupled plasma optical emission spectrometry[79] and 96ppm (1mmole/L) OSA after incubating for one week[30].

Silicade as a Synthetic OSA Rich Silica Water Supplement

Making silicon rich water weekly at home is easy and much less expensive and more sustainable than purchasing water bottled in Fiji or Malaysia. I call this water "Silicade" and there is a You Tube Video on how to make it at **"Silica Water – How to Make it at Home"**. Silicade provides 124ppm of dissolved silica to lower your body-burden of aluminum. Silicade preparation requires only two ingredients and a set of small measuring spoons that in the U.S.A. can be purchased online and shipped to your home. Silicade can be stored indefinitely in the dark like Fiji water. The chemicals to make Silicade store well and should be kept out of children's reach:

- **Low Alkalinity Hydrous Sodium Silicate:** a hydrous powder available online from ChemicalStore.com. The powder is safer and easier to measure than the liquid form but has the same ratio of 3.22 SiO_2 to Na_2O. The powder has a as a purity of 99.5% and a formula of $SiO_2[Na_2O]_{1/3.22}$ H_2O (18.5% water) Mw of 97.25. **Only order "sodium silicate – low alkalinity". Do not order "sodium silicate – alkaline" from the ChemicalStore.com or Zchemicals.com.** This powdery chemical can be stored indefinitely in its screw-cap plastic container but slowly clumps. The clumps are easily converted back to powder with a small mortar and pestle.

  Note: This solid sodium silicate from the Chemical Store is Product G manufactured by the PQ Corporation of Valley Forge, PA. Brenntag Specialties (Telephone No. 888-926-4151) buys Product G from PQ Corporation and resells it worldwide as G Sodium Silicate product number 387721 in 50-pound bags. ChemicalStore.com and Zchemicals.com buy this product from Brenntag Specialties and sell it in 2-pound containers online.

- **Sodium Bisulfate (a.k.a. Sodium Hydrogen Sulfate):** a white powder 99.5% pure of micro-prills (i.e., very small pellets) from Professor Fullwood of LoudWolf Ltd. is available from Amazon. **Note:** both optional calcium chloride and magnesium chloride are available from the same source.

- **Mini Measuring Spoon Set:** Norpro 3061D from Dine Company Online. Currently priced under $4 without shipping. Three measuring spoons come attached to a single ring. Only the dash (1/8 of a teaspoon) and smidgen (1/32 of a teaspoon) are used for Silicade preparation. In order to avoid accidental use of the wrong measuring spoon, remove the pinch from the ring. **Note: in the early 2000's some companies, such as Norpro and Dine, began defining and accurately calibrating the dash and smidgen measuring spoons as precise fractions of a teaspoon. Do not use antique dash and smidgen measuring spoons as they may not be correctly calibrated.**

- **Spatula:** Any small spatula with a straight-edge works to level the contents of the measuring spoons prior to addition.

Detailed Instructions with Options for Making Silicade

By following these detailed instructions, you can prepare a gallon of Silicade or just follow the "Short Recipe for Silicade" that follows after these detailed instructions:

1) A level dash and two level smidgens (3/16 of a teaspoon, 600mg) of hydrous powdered sodium silicate is placed in a Pyrex glass measuring cup. Add 1/8 cup of tap water and bring to boiling in the microwave or on the stove, and let boil for 30sec. This powder contains 99.5% water soluble sodium silicate monohydrate and a maximum of 0.5% of water insoluble materials, as required by the American Waterworks Standard B104-98 for adding sodium silicate to drinking water[23].
   Note: Do not heat to boiling more than 1/8 cup of tap water as more water will lower the pH making the sodium silicate less soluble.

2) The hot water with dissolved sodium silicate is immediately diluted to one gallon (3.785 liters) with cold tap water resulting in a 1.32 mM/liter (127ppm) solution of pH 9.8 OSA.

3) One level dash (1/8 of a teaspoon, 0.83 gr, 6.9 mM) of sodium bisulfate is added to the solution of OSA and dissolved with stirring in order to acidify the solution to pH 4 to 5. **Optionally**, if tap water is more basic than pH 8.5, use a pH meter while slowly adding a little more sodium bisulfate in order to lower the pH to 4.0-5.0. A pH 7.0 standard solution is recommended for periodic calibration of the pH meter.

4) The clear colorless acidic solution of OSA is further purified by filtering through a Brita pitcher style filter resulting in OSA at a pH of 4.4. This removes impurities added with sodium silicate and sodium bisulfate.

5) Two level smidgens of sodium bicarbonate (a.k.a. baking soda) are added and dissolved with stirring in the gallon of filtered OSA, resulting in Silicade with a pH of 6.5, a TDS of 285 at 25°C, and less than 2mcg/L labile aluminum. Each quart of freshly-made Silicade contains 37.4mg of dissolved silicon as 127ppm of monomeric (OSA). If allowed to stand for 72 hours at 25°C, the OSA concentration increases to 146ppm.

6) **Optionally make Silicade Plus Calcium,** if tap water is low in calcium, add two level dashes of calcium chloride flakes or prills (840mg 36% calcium) 99% pure from Loudwolf/Amazon. This will increase the calcium level by 80 ppm, the TDS to 450 at 25°C, and the pH to 6.6 in a gallon of Silicade + Ca. Labile aluminum in calcium enriched Silicade is less than 2mcg/L. Calcium at concentrations greater than or equal to 75ppm have a significant protective effect on cognition[433]. Optionally in order to increase magnesium by 20ppm add a dash of magnesium chloride hexahydrate ($\geq$98% purity) from LoudWolf/Amazon. **Optionally make Sparkling Silicade** – Carbonating Silicade will result in a pH 4.5 sparkling beverage.

Drink 3 to 4 cups of Silicade a day around meal times in order to provide a total of 30.5 to 40.7mg of silicon as monomeric OSA. This is 7.9 to 12.3 times the 3.3mg of silicon that when consumed as OSA per day was observed to lower the frequency of AD[118]. Silicade contains 127-146ppm of OSA and in the U.S.A. 160ppm of OSA (i.e., 100ppm of SiO_2) is generally recognized as safe in drinking water[22].

Short Recipe for Silicade

Ingredients needed:

- *Sodium Silicate*
- *Sodium Bisulfate*
- *Baking Soda (sodium bicarbonate)*

Tools needed:

- *Dash measuring spoon = 1/8 tsp*
- *Smidgen measuring spoon = 1/32 tsp*
- *1 cup Pyrex measuring cup*
- *1 gallon measuring container*
- *Brita filter - pitcher style*
- *Spatula for leveling*
- *Stirring utensil*

Steps:

1. Add 1 level dash & 2 level smidgens of sodium silicate to a one-cup Pyrex container

2. Add 1/8 cup of tap water to the one-cup Pyrex measuring container

3. Heat the contents of the Pyrex measuring cup to boiling and boil for at least 30 seconds

4. Dilute immediately with a small amount of unheated tap water

5. Pour all the contents of the Pyrex measuring cup into a 1-gallon container

6. Fill the 1-gallon container with unheated tap water to the 1 gallon mark on the container

7. Add 1 level dash of sodium bisulfate to the 1-gallon container

8. Stir the mixture thoroughly and then filter the mixture through a Brita filter pitcher

9. After filtering, add 2 level smidgens of baking soda (sodium bicarbonate) to the mixture

10. Stir Silicade to dissolve the baking soda

11. Enjoy the health benefits of drinking Silicade!

Silicade can be stored indefinitely in the dark at room temperature or in a refrigerator.

A You Tube video of this procedure is at: "Silica Water – How to Make it at Home"

Why This Recipe Works

The goal of this recipe for orthosilicic acid (OSA) in drinking water is to use an easily measured solid silica powder and an acidic microprill that are commercially available online and shipped to anyone, not just chemical laboratories. Both of these chemicals are high purity (i.e., 99.5%).

- **Solubilize sodium silicate:** Boiling powdered sodium silicate for 30 seconds in an eighth of a cup of tap water keeps the pH high enough (i.e., pH = 13) to solubilize silicate[434-436].

- **Neutralize to form OSA and prevent polymerization:** In order to form OSA and other silica species in equilibrium with OSA[489] and to prevent OSA polymerization[435-437], immediately dilute the basic (i.e., pH=13) OSA solution to a gallon with tap water and then immediately **render the solution non-hazardous** by acidifying the solution to pH 4 to 5 with the solid acid sodium bisulfate. A 1.32M OSA solution is well below OSA's saturation level in water (i.e., 2-3mM) but requires 72 hours to fully stabilize rising from 127ppm immediately after preparation to 146ppm[174]. Polymerization of OSA has been observed at neutral pH only well above OSA's 200ppm saturation level[435-437].

- **Remove Aluminum:** For optimal aluminum removal acidify the OSA solution with sodium bisulfate to pH 4.0 to 5.0 and then filter through a Brita pitcher style filter (OB03)[174]. A significant portion (i.e., 98.5%) of the labile aluminum introduced in tap water is removed[174,175]. This Brita filter is a combined activated carbon and weak cation exchange resin that removes cations like aluminum but does not remove OSA[174]. If the tap water used for Silicade is between pH 6.5 to 8.5, as per EPA's secondary drinking water standard, then after acidification, filtration, and bicarbonate addition Silicade will be pH 6.5.

- **Optionally add Calcium and/or Magnesium:** Have your tap water checked and if it is low in calcium and/or magnesium, add supplemental calcium and/or magnesium to Silicade. The Brita filter reduces calcium and magnesium in Quabbin tap water by one half[175]. Drinking water with calcium at levels of 80mg and magnesium at levels of 20 ppm has been found to be optimal for good health[438]. This may be due to calcium and magnesium competing with aluminum for absorption by the gut[433]. Calcium catalyzes the polymerization of OSA but only at pH greater than 8[18,19]. Silicade + Ca is pH 6.6 and at this pH OSA in Silicade + Ca is primarily a non-polymeric monomer[174,439].

Chapter 7- Safety of OSA Ingestion and Handling of Sodium Silicate

A safe strategy for OSA supplementation is to start with 1 cup a day for adults or ½ cup a day for children and work up to drinking 3 to 4 cups over a 9 to 12-hour period during the day of either silica rich mineral water or homemade Silicade (see Appendix I and Chapter 6). Mothers should drink OSA rich water prior to pregnancy and, if there are no side effects, continue drinking OSA rich water during pregnancy and while breast feeding.

Side-effects of Taking Supplemental OSA Rich Silica Water

Most people do not have side-effects. But starting on OSA rich water should be done slowly with lower doses while checking for side-effects. Side-effects include: headache, due to an increase of aluminum in both urine and blood. Supplemental OSA temporarily enhances aluminum levels in the urine as shown in Figure 7b[77]. Side-effects can also include fatigue and irritability, likely due to aluminum inhibiting glycolysis[442]. Glycolysis is the body's way of getting energy from carbohydrates. These side-effects may be more pronounced in those people who have accumulated more aluminum or are routinely consuming too much aluminum. Therefore, eliminating sources of aluminum from the diet and OSA supplementation are recommended (see Appendix I and II). Taking OSA in small doses during the day will lessen side-effects.

Safety of OSA Ingestion

It is safe to ingest dissolved silicates, such as OSA, at concentrations well below the saturation level (i.e., less than 200ppm of OSA) in order to ensure that they will not become supersaturated and crystallize in the kidney lumen.

OSA is the monomeric bioavailable form of dissolved silica commonly found in rivers, lakes, aquifers, and drinking waters around the world[435]. "Dissolved silica from commercial soluble silicates is indistinguishable from natural dissolved silica."[191]. The amount of OSA in drinking water varies widely depending upon the source (see Chapter 5). In the U.S.A. 160 ppm of dissolved silicates, such as OSA, are generally recognized as safe (GRAS) in drinking water by the FDA[22]. The adequate intake of water per day is 3 liters for men and 2.3 liters for women.

This level of water intake corresponds to a maximum safe level of OSA intake per day of 480mg for men and 368mg for women. Therefore, drinking 3 to 4 cups of supplemental silica water each day containing a total of 90 to 138mg of OSA (equivalent to 26.5 to 40.5mg of Si) is well below the GRAS level for dissolved silicates (see Table 33).

Ingesting OSA near or above the saturation level (i.e., 200ppm) can result in kidney stones (a.k.a. nephrolithiasis) in dogs but almost never in humans. There is one report of kidney stones resulting from a silicate salt incorrectly labeled as SiO_2 and used as an inactive ingredient (a.k.a. excipient) in several over-the-counter drugs such as Uncaria Tomentosa, Digestive Advantage, and FlexProtein supplements[441].

Safety of Low Bioavailability, Untested, and Zeolite Containing Products

Choline stabilized OSA, sold as **Biosil**, is a combination of 200mg of choline with 10mg of silicon as silicate. There is a 70% greater risk of lethal prostate cancer with high (500mg/day) choline diets[430]. Note that The European Food Safety Authority therefore recommends that liquid choline stabilized OSA be taken at a maximum dose of 10 drops equivalent to 10 mg of silicon as silicate complexed with 200mg of choline per day[431,432]. Also, since the use of Biosil in children has not been studied, the Biosil Corporation does not recommend it to be used in children under age seven.

Jarrow Formulas have developed a product called **JarroSil** that contains molecular clusters of stabilized silicic acid. JarroSil is less expensive per ounce than BioSil, but JarroSil only contains 0.4 mg of silicon as silicic acid per drop as compared with 1 mg of silicon per drop in BioSil. No tests have been published on the safety or JarroSil or the bioavailability of OSA in JarroSil.

In Europe a company, Silicium Laboratories, is promoting a non-natural silica as a supplement called **monomethyl silanetriol (MMST)**. MMST in water is absorbed by the gut and made 64% bioavailable when dissolved in alcohol free beer[79]. There is no data showing that MMST facilitates elimination of aluminum from the body. In addition, the lack of toxicity data on MMST makes it impossible to recommend MMST at the present time.

Zeolites are microporus alumininosilicate minerals that are both produced on large scale industrially and also occur in nature. Depending on how they are made, they can exist in different 3-D frameworks. Zeolites when inhaled can cause lung cancer. Zeolites when taken orally decrease immune activity in the body, facilitate the removal of essential minerals from the gut, dissolve aluminum into the gut, and decrease the effectiveness of some oral medications. Therefore, zeolites can't be recommended as an oral supplement.

Clinoptilolite Zeolite as nanoparticles has been commercially promoted under the tradename **TRS** for toxic metal detox. However, oral administration of clinoptilolite zeolite has **not** been shown to facilitate elimination of aluminum. In fact, it has been shown that there is a net release of dissolved aluminum from clinoptilolite in simulated human gastric fluid[482]. Accumulation of zeolites in the body during long term use of TRS is a health risk as dissolution of slowly accumulating zeolites will increase aluminum exposure to organs of the body, such as the brain. This is evidenced by the amount of aluminum in urine being proportional to the number of years ingesting clinoptilolite zeolites. For example: no zeolite ingestion 7.5ppm, 1-3 years of zeolite ingestion 15.3ppm, and 6-13 years of zeolite ingestion 39.9ppm of aluminum in urine[483].

Simulated digestion of clinoptilolite zeolite as particles larger than nanoparticles has been shown to result in a net release of dissolved aluminum[482] in spite of the proven ability of clinoptilolite zeolite to absorb aluminum[484]. The researchers point out that this loss of material during gastric digestion "might be related to the possible dissolution process of aluminosilicates at the surface layer …"[482]. The smaller the size of the zeolite particle - the greater the surface layer and the faster aluminum is dissolved from the zeolite. This is disturbing because a 1 nanometer sized particle has over 10,000 times more surface area than larger particles used in the simulated digestion study[482]. Therefore, it can be predicted that much more aluminum will dissolve after ingestion of nanoparticles as compared with larger particles of zeolite.

This data has convinced the FDA that clinoptilolite zeolites should **not** be generally regarded as safe (GRAS) when ingested by animals. In a May 4th 2018 letter from Dr. David Edwards, the Director of the Division of Animal Feeds for the FDA, to a producer of animal feed containing clinoptilolite zeolites, Dr. Edwards said their animal feeds are **not** GRAS because the use of clinoptilolite zeolites in animal feed **"… could cause potential excess levels of aluminum … in some species"**[485].

Interactions of Epsom Salt baths with Drinking OSA

Aluminum accumulation in the body inhibits both the methylation and transsulfuration pathways[100,101]. This results in higher-than-normal levels of homocysteine and lower than normal levels of SAM, reduced glutathione, and **sulfate** that are biomarkers for autism[1,455]. Some people have recommended Epsom salt (i.e., magnesium sulfate) baths as a way to supplement sulfate in those with autism.

The concentration of sulfate increases in the urine by 50 to 75% for at least 24 hours after a 12-minute bath in a dilute 1% (i.e., 1 gr. per 100cc) Epsom salt solution[456]. For instance, the mean pre-bath sulfate level in the urine of 19 people (14-64 years of age, 10 males and 9 females) was 60ppm with a mean post-bath sulfate level of 105ppm[456].

Also, the concentration of magnesium increases in the blood due to Epson salt baths. Blood magnesium rises on average 9% after a 12-minute Epson salt bath and blood magnesium rises 35% after 7 days of daily bathing for 12-minutes per day in an Epson salt bath[456]. Higher than normal levels of magnesium in the blood of children is called hypermagnesemia that can inhibit the enzyme Na^+/K^+ ATPase that is responsible for potassium ion transport into the intracellular space in neurons and muscle[457]. Aluminum also inhibits Na^+/K^+ ATPase[490]. This inhibition by either or both magnesium and aluminum also causes inhibition of choline reuptake and cholinergic disruption as is fully explained on rung 17 in my book "Finding a Cause and Potential Cures for Alzheimer's Disease".

Therefore, Epson salt baths may stifle the benefits seen in drinking OSA rich silica water to facilitate elimination of aluminum. The following anecdotal information supports this conclusion:

"My 9 year old son has severe autism … After previous Epsom Salt baths he has been fine, although no real obvious improvements. However, the first one I decided to give him since he started drinking silica water 9 weeks ago stopped the silica water improvements in their tracks and he resorted back to his pre-silica-water-self for example lots of hand/arm movements, repeating words rather than asking for things, less calm, and obsessive behavior". September 2018

Handling of Sodium Silicate

One of the questions repeatedly asked is: "Can sodium silicate cause silicosis?" First of all silicosis is an occupational lung disease caused by inhaling crystalline silica dust less than 10 micrometers in diameter. There are seven different forms of crystalline silica and they all consist of water insoluble silicon dioxide (a.k.a. SiO_2). Sodium silicate ($Na_2Si_{3.22}O_{7.44}$) is the sodium salt of water-soluble silicic acid ($Si(OH)_4$). **Sodium silicate is not silicon dioxide and therefore inhalation of sodium silicate powder does not cause silicosis.**

Sodium silicate when dissolved in water is basic (pH greater than 7) and if not neutralized with an acid, such as sodium bisulfate, could cause skin and eye irritation. This same type of irritation is felt when soap gets into the eyes while bathing, as soap is also basic. In order to prevent irritation, avoid skin and eye contact with sodium silicate as a powder or as a non-neutralized solution in water. **If experiencing skin or eye irritation while handling sodium silicate, then rinse the exposed area with excess water until the irritation subsides.**

Hydrous low alkalinity sodium silicate powder as purchased from the ChemicalStore.com is comprised of crystalline clusters that are not small enough to be suspended in air as a dust. In addition, powdered sodium silicate has virtually no vapor pressure at room temperature and does not evaporate or sublime into air even in boiling water. At above 1,100°C the vapor pressure of sodium silicate is still 20,000-fold less than water at room temperature[440]. So, for these reasons **no special respiratory protection is required when measuring sodium silicate powder or boiling sodium silicate powder in water.**

Keep all chemicals out of the reach of children.

Conclusion – Resiliency for Healthy Longevity

As the world changes so must we in order to survive. Resiliency is the ability to adjust to these changes. We entered the Aluminum Age in 1888 when Karl Joseph Bayer developed a process to refine aluminum from bauxite ore. This process opened a Pandora's Box of low-cost aluminum products that have changed our life for the better and our health for the worse. Our collective survival requires that we all become **individually resilient** to our increasing exposure to aluminum. By taking clues from plants and animals that are resilient to aluminum exposure and by studying the resiliency of those living in the longevity regions of the world, the secret has been discovered of how to prevent and heal from aluminum toxicity in the Aluminum Age:

Drinking OSA rich silica water can reduce aluminum accumulation in our bodies and prevent 7 terminal diseases in which aluminum is a causal factor: Alzheimer's, heart disease, stroke, cancer, multiple sclerosis, osteoporosis, and Parkinson's. Also drinking OSA rich silica water can improve the odds of conception and lower the risk of autism and seizures and even heal from autism and seizures.

This technological breakthrough was made by a group of dedicated researchers who have spent the last two decades making the following important discoveries:

- Silica water taken orally facilitates the elimination of aluminum from the body, in both urine and sweat, and prevents aluminum accumulation in the body.
- There are six longevity regions in the world where people live significantly longer than those living just outside the longevity regions.
- Silica, as OSA, is at higher-than-normal concentrations in the drinking water of all six longevity regions.
- There are a number of diseases whose incidence is increasing in lock-step with worldwide aluminum production.
- In all cases aluminum accumulation has been shown to be a causal factor of these diseases.

We are confronted with the rising incidence of a number of terminal **mismatch diseases**. In these cases, our Paleolithic bodies are mismatched to our changing environment by being inadequately adapted to the aluminum age. Since these diseases cause mortality and reduce the longevity of populations around the world, by drinking OSA rich silica water and eating OSA rich vegetables the risk of these diseases can be reduced, resulting in healthy longevity. The information in this book provides a mechanism for both individual and cultural adaption. **Individual and cultural resiliency** gives us the strength to adapt by taking action and supplementing our drinking water with OSA rich silica water and eating OSA rich vegetables. In addition, we can take steps to lower our aluminum ingestion and that of our children.

Not everyone has the necessary **individual resiliency** to adapt their diet and lifestyle for self-protection from mismatch diseases. A case in point is Professor Louis F. Fieser. For the fall semester at Harvard in 1965 I had high expectations of taking Professor Fieser's Chem. 20 course on organic chemistry. To my great disappointment a substitute teacher explained Professor Fieser had been diagnosed with lung cancer, had a lung removed, and would not be teaching Chem. 20. The ironic part of the story is that in 1962 Professor Fieser had served as one of the ten men on the U.S. Surgeon General's advisory committee that issued the influential 1964 report concluding smoking is a causal factor of lung cancer. Even though he agreed with committee's conclusion, he did not stop smoking four packs a day until his lung was removed.

This book is a **handbook for individual resiliency** in the aluminum age as it contains the following information:

- Natural mineral waters of the world that contain OSA greater than 49ppm listed by country
- Vegetables containing OSA listed in order of their OSA content
- Beer types of the world that contain high levels of OSA are ranked by type
- Complete instructions for Silicade an inexpensive homemade synthetic OSA rich silica water
- Daily sources of aluminum listed with the amount of aluminum per serving
- Plots of increasing incidence of mismatch diseases versus increasing aluminum production
- The science behind why aluminum is a likely causal factor of these mismatch diseases
- The science behind why drinking silica water facilitates the elimination of aluminum
- Anecdotal information of recovery from autism, seizures, and MS with silica water & OSA

A perfect example **of individual resiliency** is that mothers should drink OSA rich water prior to pregnancy and, if there are no side effects, continue drinking OSA rich water during pregnancy and while breast feeding. We can also display our **individual resiliency** and give our children silica water for at least several months after vaccinations with aluminum containing vaccines.

You may wonder why your doctor hasn't mentioned drinking OSA rich water on a regular basis for healthy longevity. The information presented in this book is primarily the result of recent research and your doctor is likely unaware of this research. The pharmaceutical industry is the primary source of information on new drugs. Silica water is not a pharmaceutical drug and therefore will not be promoted by drug companies for prescription by doctors. Medical training and traditions can be counter to the adoption of new innovations. Your choice is to wait for medical practice to catch up with research or you can start drinking silica water and see for yourself.

I hope this book becomes a handbook for **cultural resiliency** as there is nothing stopping any community from becoming a longevity region by just adding OSA to their drinking water. There is already an American Water Works Standard B404-98 for adding OSA (i.e., sodium silicate) to community drinking water for corrosion control[23]. Why not add OSA to community drinking water for both corrosion control and public health?

Also, we should demonstrate our **cultural resiliency** and demand that aluminum not be added to food. In addition, we should demand that if aluminum is found to be naturally present in food, the concentration of aluminum should be printed on the product label.

Also, we should demonstrate our **cultural resiliency** and demand that aluminum not be added to vaccines. In addition, all vaccine schedules should be changed to postpone vaccination with aluminum containing vaccines until children are 3 months or older. Finally, we should work to avoid vaccinating children with vaccines that both contain aluminum and are not lifesaving vaccines.

Appendix I – Bottled Silica Waters of the World

This following list of silica waters of the world was provided by Paul Watling and http://www.finewaters.com/bottled-waters-of-the-world. When purchasing silica water be sure to check the label as silica levels can be subject to change.

Table 34. International Silica Waters – With Greater than 49 ppm OSA			
Country of Origin	Brand	Silica ppm	OSA ppm
Australia	Three Bays	56	89.6
Australia	Cottonwood Springs	57	91
Austria	Gussinger	41.6	66.6
Austria	Waldquelle	41.1	65.8
Austria	Long Life – Bad Radkersberg	97.9	162.9
China	Tang Emperor Mineral Spring Water	107.1	171.4
China	Leishan	62.2	99.5
China	Dukang	50	80
China	Sino Fillipino	45.6	72.9
China	Lugmen Shan	39.5	63.2
China	Kosnitval	39.5	63.2
China	Xiao Xi	39.5	63.2
China	Kesal	35.6	57
China	Juifeng	33.8	54.1
Croatia	Studenac	41.1	65.8
Czech Republic	Magnesia	61.1	97.8
Fiji	Fiji Water	93	148.8 [146]
Fiji	Aqua Pacific	61	97.6
Fiji	Savu	33	52.8
France	Arie	83.3	133.3
France	Le Salvetat	72.2	115.5
France	Arcens	49.9	79.8
France	Luciole	42.3	67.7
France	Puits St George	36.9	59
France	Chambon / Source Montfras	36.2	57.9
France	Mont-Dore	33.7	53.9
France	Volvic	31.7	50.7 [51]

Table 34. International Silica Waters - continued			
Country of Origin	Brand	Silica ppm	OSA ppm
Germany	Vulkani Heilwasser	83.5	133.6
Germany	St Linus Heilvasser	58.9	92.2
Germany	Dunaris	54.9	87.8
Germany	Hirschquelle	53.9	86.2
Germany	Konig Otto Sprudel	50	80
Germany	Wildsber Quelle	40.9	65.4
Germany	Gerolsteiner	40.2	64.3
Germany	Teinacher	40	64
Germany	Tonissteiner	35.4	56.6
Germany	Wittenseer Quelle	33.4	53.4
Germany	Eifel Stil	33.3	53.3
Hungary	Kristalyviz	52.8	84.5
Hungary	Aqua Mathias	46.6	74.6
Hungary	383 the Kopjary Water	31	49.6
Italy	Egeria	108.5	173.6
Italy	Gaudianella	105.1	168.2
Italy	Claudia	103	164.8
Italy	Appia	101	161.6
Italy	Ninfa	99.2	158.7
Italy	Koccafina	89	142.4
Italy	H2Opera	86.6	138.6
Italy	Ferrarelle	81.1	129.8
Italy	Acqua di Nepi	80	128
Italy	Santagata	72.2	115.5
Italy	Natia	68.8	110.1
Italy	S Maria Degli Angeli	65.7	105.1
Italy	Toka	63.3	101.3
Italy	Tione	63.2	101.1
Italy	Funte Fria	48.3	77.3
Italy	Fiuggi Aqua Minerale Naturale	48	76.8
Italy	Sole	40	64
Japan	Fine	81.5	130.4
Lithuania	Vytautas	38	60.8
Malaysia	Acilis	55.2	88.3
Malaysia	Spritzer	43	69
Malaysia	Langkawi Pure	84.9	135.8 [133]

Table 34. International Silica Waters - continued			
Country of Origin	**Brand**	**Silica ppm**	**OSA ppm**
New Zealand	Nakd	81.5	130.4
New Zealand	Te Waihau	77.8	124.5
New Zealand	Antipodes	76	121.6
New Zealand	Kiwaii	75	120
Peru	Socosani	64	102.4
Portugal	Lombadas	74.4	119
Portugal	Pedras Salgadas	71.4	114.2
Portugal	Pedras	62	99.2
Portugal	Salus Vidago	52.4	83.8
Portugal	Carvalhelhos	39.1	62.6
Portugal	Aguas de Bem Saude	31.1	49.8
Russia	Navoterskaya Tselebraya	45.5	72.8
Slovenia	ROI 86	86	137.6
Slovenia	Rogaska	61.1	97.8
Slovakia	Santovka	46.2	73.9
Slovenia	Radenska	35	56
Spain	Pinalito	135.3	216.5
Spain	Firgas	112.1	179.4
Spain	Malavella	77.2	123.5
Spain	San Narciso	71.9	115
Spain	Aguacassa	70	112
Spain	Agua de Sousas	61.1	97.8
Spain	Fuenteror	56.6	90.6
Spain	Fontecelta	40.7	65.1
Spain	Aigua de Vilajuija Water	40	64
Spain	Fuensanta	33.3	53.3
Spain	Fonteide	31.2	49.9
United States	Starkey Spring Water	58.9	94.2 [93]
United States	Hawaiian Springs Bottled Water	37	59.2
United States	Wiakeia Hawaiian Volcano Water	44	70.4
Vietnam	Thianh Tan	54.8	87.7

Note: the ppm's in brackets are test results of the author's 2022 Coradin's blue assay for OSA[29,174]

Beer as a Source of OSA

Commercial bottled beer contains high levels of OSA ranging from 22 to 192ppm of OSA. Beer made from the grist of barley contains more silica than beer made from the grist of wheat (see Table 23). Even though hops contain more silica than grains, the amount of hops used in beer is relatively small compared to grain. Therefore, most of the silica is added by grain. During brewing most of the silica remains with the spent grains. But with aggressive treatment of the liquid extracted from the mashing process much of this silica is released as OSA that survives into beer[443]. For average OSA levels in different types of beer see Table 35.

Table 35. OSA Content of Commercial Beers[443]			
Category	Average OSA ppm	Range of OSA ppm	Types Tested
IPA	140	89 - 189	15
Pale Ale	124	57 - 172	18
Ales	112	38 - 189	67
Lagers	81	34 - 192	36
Wheat	64	49 - 80	7
Light Lagers	58	48 - 80	5
Non-alcoholic	55	22 - 87	6

Each beer was degassed and tested for silicon (Si) by inductively coupled plasma atomic spectrometry[443]. All readings for silicon were multiplied by 3.4 to get OSA levels in beer.

Avoid Drinking from Aluminum Cans and Bottles

Beers and soft drinks sold in aluminum cans should be avoided whenever possible. The enamel coating on the inside of the can contains pinholes that allow beer to corrode the aluminum can adding aluminum to beer[1]. This corrosion adds both neurotoxic aluminum and, for some of us, a metallic taste to the beer. Approximately 30% of people can taste high levels of aluminum.

Appendix II – Daily Sources of Aluminum

Aluminum can be accumulated in the body by oral ingestion, inhaled as vapor, or injected as an adjuvant in a vaccine. Orally ingested aluminum is preferentially accumulated in the brain, bone, liver, spleen, and kidney of rats[64] and the brain, breast, retinal, and ovarian tissues of mice[444]. Aluminum has also been shown to accumulate in the brains of humans[266]. Inhaled aluminum is preferentially accumulated in the brain of rats via the olfactory nerve[67]. Aluminum in tobacco and cannabis (as much as 0.37% and 0.4% by weight respectively) is volatilized during smoking and is absorbed by the lungs during both active and passive second-hand exposure to smoke[445].

Avoid products with any ingredient on a label than includes the words: alum, alumina, aluminum, or bauxite.

Daily sources of aluminum are listed in Table 36 with the highest indicated with a "*" :

Table 36. Daily Sources of Aluminum[1,174,445-450]			
Source of Aluminum (Al)	**Examples**	**Aluminum (mcg)**	**Safer Alternatives**
Al Cookware*	Pots, Pans, Calderos, &	775/liter H_2O -	Stainless Steel
	Dutch Ovens	350 °F for 1hr.	Cast Iron
			Porcelain - Ceramic
			Non-stick Thermalon
	Aluminum Foil	60,000-220,000	Non-stick Al Foil
		Per Kg of beef	Parchment Paper
		baked 1-3hr.	Plastic Wrap Under Foil
Antacids*	Aluminum Hydroxide:		Calcium Carbonate:
	Equate - Liquid	138,330/tsp	CVS Natural Antacid
	Maalox - Liquid	138,750/tsp	Aluminum= 90mcg/tablet
	Mylanta - Tablets	69,170/tablet	
	Mylanta - Liquid	170,910/tsp	
	Gelusil - Tablets	69,170/tablet	
	Magnesium Aluminum		
	Silicate - Veegum		
Antiperspirants	Alum, Bauxite, &	4/use absorbed	Arm & Hammer Essentials
	Aluminum Chlorohydrate		Schimdts

Table 36. Daily Sources of Aluminum - Continued			
Source of Aluminum (Al)	**Examples**	**Aluminum (mcg)**	**Safer Alternatives**
Baking Powder*	Acid = Alum:		Acid = Cream of Tartar:
	Davis	48,600/tsp	Homemade Baking Pdr.:
	"Aluminum Free":		Cream of Tartar 2 tsp
	Rumford	790/tsp	Baking Soda 1 tsp
	Market Pantry	930/tsp	Corn Starch 1 tsp
	Trader Joe's	>1,000/tsp	Aluminum < 4mcg/tsp
	Whole Foods 365	>1,000/tsp	
Coffee Makers*	Aluminum Containing:		Non-aluminum Containing:
	Drip Style:		Drip Style:
	Black & Decker 1050	37-264/liter	BUNN Speed Brew
	Cuisinart DCC-450	52/liter	Jura Compresso MG900
	Cuisinart DCC-1200	182/liter	Nespresso + cups C110
	Percolator Style:		Keurig K90
	Presto 0281104	82/liter	Krups Moka Brew
	Hawthorn 3424	260/liter	Percolator Style:
			Farberware FCP-412
			Farberware FCP-240A
Colorants*	Aluminum Lakes:		No Aluminum Lakes:
	Kellog Cherry Poptart	1,110/serving	Natural Food Colorants
	Marsh Green Cookie	154/serving	See Color Kitchen's
	Cupcakes:		
	Hostess Orange	470/serving	
	Betty Crocker Blue	84/serving	
	Betty Crocker Red	3,470/serving	
	Okedoke Chessy	420/serving	
	Combos	350/serving	
	Hamburger Helper	1,040/cup	
	Scalloped Potatoes	380/cup	
	M&M Milk Chocolate	2,950/48 pieces	
	M&M Peanuts	1,410/15 pieces	
	Skittles Original	3,320/61 pieces	
	Reese's Pieces	660/51 pieces	
	Rainbow Nerds	370/Tbls	
	Sprees	230/8 pieces	
	Jawbreakers:		
	Red	130/3 pieces	
	Orange	50/3 pieces	
	Purple	70/3 pieces	
	Green	50/3 pieces	
	Yellow	27/3 pieces	

Table 36. Daily Sources of Aluminum - Continued			
Source of Aluminum (Al)	**Examples**	**Aluminum (mcg)**	**Safer Alternatives**
Cosmetics	Aluminum Containing		Non-aluminum Containing
	Sun Screens & Blocks		Zinc Oxide Sun Screens
	Lipstick		
	Styptic Pencil		
Drinking Water	Tap Water- Alum Treated	179/liter avg.	Tap Water- Brita Filtered
	Bottled Water:		Bottled Water:
	AquaFina	5/liter	Fiji Water 0 mcg/liter
	Eska	5/liter	Poland Spring 0 mcg/liter
	Evian	7/liter	Starkey Water 0 mcg/liter
	Perrier	13/liter	Volvic 0 mcg/liter
	San Pellagrino	23/liter	
	Alumina for Fluoride	1,000/ppm of F	Bone Char for Fluoride
	Removal		Removal
E-Cigarettes	10% Al on Woven Tube	4.4/15 puffs	Avoid E-Cigarettes
	in Core of E-Cigarette		
Food*	Contains Baking Powder:		Use Aluminum Free B.P.
	Brownies		
	Cakes		
	Corn Bread		
	Cupcakes		
	Donuts		
	Biscotti		
	Biscuits		
	Muffins		
	Pancakes		
	Scones		
	Tortillas		
	Waffles		
	Fried Chicken		
	Chicken McNuggets		
	Food Containing Alum:		
	Cheese Shredded		
	Some Mt Olive Pickles		
	Some Salt		

Table 36. Daily Sources of Aluminum - Continued

Source of Aluminum (Al)	Examples	Aluminum (mcg)	Safer Alternatives
Pharmaceuticals*	Al as Active Ingredient:		
	Ascriptin Buff. Aspirin		CVS Buffered Aspirin
	Aluminum as Colorant:		
	Bayer LowDoseAspirin		Walgreen LowDoseAspirin
	Citrucel Caplets		
	Levothyroxine		50mcg pill is white
	Musinex 12 Hour		
	Aluminum for Anticaking		
	Centrum Multivitamins		
	Aluminum as Astringent:		
	Domboro		Use Epson Salts
	Canker Sore Powder		
	Aluminum as Zeolites		Use silica water and
			Selenomethionine
	Aluminum in Seizure		Use silica water
	Medications		
	Clobazam		
	Lamictal		
Pigments	Used for Tattooing		
	Carmine / Carmine Lake	5.5% by Wt. Al	
	EU food additive E120		
	(a.k.a. Cochinal)		
Shampoos	Dry Shampoo		
	Some Dandruff Shampoo		
Soaps	Dove Orig Beauty Cream		
	EnviroKlenz Odor		
	Neutralizing Soap		
Spices	Alum*	5.7% by Wt. Al	Dispose of all Alum
Tobacco*	Aluminum Accumulators	0.4% by Wt. Al	Don't Smoke
& Cannabis*			

Appendix III – Vaccines That Contain Aluminum

Vaccines contain aluminum as an adjuvant. When injected this aluminum is 23% to 73% bioavailable as opposed to ingested aluminum in foods and water that is only 0.2% bioavailable (i.e., the amount that gets into the blood stream and is accumulated or excreted as urine.) Aluminum that is used as an adjuvant in the vaccine is released slowly over at least 28 days after the vaccination[451]. Some of the aluminum adjuvants injected as vaccines in rabbits have been found to be accumulated in their brains[451].

Note that depending upon manufacturer the amount of aluminum for a given vaccine can vary by a factor of approximately 2. When possible, ask for the lower dose of aluminum:

- Daptacel 330mcg and Infanrix 625mcg

- Quadracel 330mcg and Kinrix 600mcg

- Engerix 250mcg and Recombivax 500mcg

- Gardisil 225mcg and Gardasil 9 500mcg

Table 37. Vaccines that Contain Aluminum	
Vaccine	**Aluminum Content (mcg/dose)**
Daptacel (DTaP – Diptheria, Tetanus, Pertussis)	330
Infanrix (DTaP)	625
Kinrix (DTaP + Polio)	600
Pediarix (DTaP + Polio + Hepatitis B)	850
Pentacel (DTaP + Polio + Haemophilus influenza B)	330
Quadracel (DTaP + Polio)	330
PedvaxHIB (Haemophilus influenza B)	225
Havrix (Hepatitis A)	250
Vaqta (Hepatitis A)	225
Twinrix (Hepatitis A and B)	450
Engerix-B (Hepatitis B)	250
Recombivax (Hepatitis B)	500
Gardasil (Human Papillomavirus / HPV)	225
Gardasil 9 (HPV)	500
Bexsero (Meningococcal B)	519
Prevnar (Pneumococcal)	125
Td (Tetanus and Diptheria)	530
Tenivac (Tetanus and Diptheria)	330
Adacel (Tdap – Tetanus and Diptheria Booster)	330
Boostrix (Tdap – Tetanus and Diptheria Booster)	390

Appendix IV – Testing for Silica in Drinking Water

In drinking water there are primarily two forms of silica: silicon dioxide and OSA. Silicon dioxide exists in water as insoluble colloidal silica particles that if orally ingested temporarily remain in the gut and are not absorbed into the blood. OSA is soluble in water up to its saturation level of 200 ppm. If OSA rich water is orally ingested approximately 50% of the dissolved OSA is absorbed from the gut into the blood making it bioavailable, unlike silicon dioxide. Only bioavailable OSA can facilitate the removal of aluminum from the body's internal organs. The silicon dioxide in drinking water taken from an aquifer in which the water has had a long residence time (i.e., many years) usually has been slowly converted with the addition of two water molecules to OSA.

Drinking water is usually analyzed for silica in one of two ways:

- **The AWWA Silica Assay:** The total amount of both silicon dioxide and OSA in drinking water is analyzed and reported as silica or SiO_2[23]. If the water contains primarily OSA, then multiplying the silica or SiO_2 concentration by 1.6 gives the OSA concentration.
- **Coradin's Silicomolybdic Spectrophotometric Blue Assay:** Only OSA and the OSA dimer are detected by a procedure that does not detect colloids of SiO_2[29]. OSA is usually reported as the OSA or $Si(OH)_4$ concentration.

The best test for OSA is Coradin's Silicomolybdic Spectrophotometric Blue Assay as it does not detect silica colloids that are not bioavailable. However, because of its simplicity, the AWWA Silica Assay is more commonly performed.

AWWA Total Silica Gravimetric Assay of Drinking Water

A drinking water sample is filtered through a medium porosity porous-porcelain filter crucible to remove suspended matter larger than 10-15 microns in size. Note that silica colloids are not removed as they are usually more than a thousand times smaller. Fifty milliliters of the filtered sample are evaporated to dryness and the solid residue of SiO_2 and OSA is treated with acid and heat (e.g., 1,200°C) dehydrating the OSA to SiO_2. The solid white water insoluble powder of impure SiO_2 is weighed and then treated with hydrofluoric acid and heated to volatilize all silicon. The remaining residue is weighed and the weight subtracted from the weight of the impure SiO_2 powder in order to calculate the total silica concentration of SiO_2 and OSA that was in the 50 ml drinking water sample.

Coradin's Silicomolybdic Blue Spectrophotometric OSA (Si(OH)$_4$) Assay

Coradin's blue silicomolybdic spectrophotometric assay is timed to detect only OSA monomer and dimer and not detect any OSA polymer or silica colloid[29]. The assay is based on the ability of silicic acid and its dimer to quickly form a heteropolyacid, silico-12-molybdic acid, in the presence of acidified heptomolybdate. The silicomolybdic acid has a detection limit of 10^{-4} mole per liter. But when reduced to the molybdenum blue complex, concentrations as low as $5x10^{-6}$ mole per liter can be accurately measured. The reducing agent used is 4-methylaminophenol sulfate (a.k.a. metol) in the presence of sodium sulfite. Added oxalic acid leads to phosphomolybdic acid breakdown preventing phosphate interference.

In order to verify accuracy, 1 ml of both 16 and 80 ppm silica water standards traceable to the U.S. National Institute of Standards and Technology (NIST) are assayed each time a series of assays are run. A linear plot of absorbance versus OSA concentration at 0 ppm 16 ppm and 80 ppm is used for quantitation of test samples. The silica standard solutions 10 ppm SiO_2 (16 ppm OSA) in water and 50 ppm of SiO_2 in water (80 ppm OSA) were obtained from the Hach Company. **In 2022, absorbance versus OSA over 80ppm OSA was shown to be nonlinear[174]. Therefore, test samples over 80ppm OSA must be diluted with distilled water to 50-80ppm OSA immediately prior to testing and results corrected mathematically for dilution.**

Solution A is made of 1.0 gram of ammonium molybdate tetrahydrate and 3 ml of concentrated hydrochloric acid both diluted to 50 ml with distilled water. This solution is stored in a polypro bottle with polypro cap at 50°F. This solution is not stable indefinitely. However, it has proved to be good for several months.

Solution B is prepared by adding 20 grams of oxalic acid, 6.67 grams of 4-methylaminophenol sulfate, 4 grams of anhydrous sodium sulfate, and 500ml of distilled water to a 1 liter volumetric Florence flask. 100 ml of concentrated sulfuric acid was slowly added and the flask was filled to 1 liter with distilled water. This solution was bottled in two glass bottles with polypro caps.

All samples were acidified to pH 3.3 prior to testing. This is the pH of the gut and is most closely related to silicic acid bioavailability.

Stepwise OSA Method

1. 1 ml of an aqueous solution of unknown silicic acid concentration is added to a 50cc beaker.

2. 15 ml of distilled water is added to the beaker.

3. To this is added 1.5 ml of solution A containing acidic ammonium molybdate tetrahydrate.

4. After 10 minutes, 7.5 ml of solution B is added to the assay solution. Solution B contains the reducing agent with oxalic acid.

5. The blue color is left to develop over 2 hours at room temperature before measuring the optical density at 810nm with a spectrophotometer versus both a 1ml distilled water blank as a "zero" and 1 ml of both NIST traceable 16 and 80ppm standards subjected to the same procedure as the 1 ml of unknown. The spectrophotometer is adjusted to read 100% transmittance with the "zero" prior to measuring each sample.

Concordance

There is agreement within experimental error of test results from the AWWA total silica analysis and Coradin's Blue OSA assay between zero and 100ppm SiO_2 (160ppm OSA).

References

I would like to thank all the researchers referenced herein for their patience and persistence in making discoveries relevant to the subjects covered in this book. Without their research and the research of those who preceded them, there would be no information on how silica water increases healthy longevity in the Aluminum Age.

1. Crouse, D.N.; Prevent, Alzheimer's, Autism, and Stroke With 7 Supplements, 7 Lifestyle Changes, and a Dissolved Mineral; Etiological Publishing (2016)
2. Poulain, M., et al.; The blue zs: areas of exceptional longevity around the world; Vienna Yearbook of Population Research; 11:87-108 (2013)
3. De Zuane, J.; Handbook of Drinking Water Quality; John Wiley & Sons; (1997)
4. City of Loma Linda; Annual Water Quality Report; PWS ID#:36100 (2015)
5. Lowell, F.W., et al.; Appraisal of ground-water quality in the Bunker Hill Basin of San Bernardion Valley, California; U.S. Geological Survey; Water-resources investigations report 88-4203 (1989)
6. The Study on Rural Development Project for the Middle Basin of Tempisque River Final Report; Table on p3-14 Guardia and Guinea Survey Points Wet and Dry Seasons: Data Source: Instituto Costarricense de Electricidad Datos de Calidad de Aguas, Sistema Hidromet, (1987-1991)
7. Karakatsanis, S., et al.; Chemical characterization of the thermal springs along the South Aegean volcanic arc and Ikaria Island; (2011)
8. Ciotoli, G., and Guerra, M.; Distribution and physico-chemical data of Italian bottled natural mineral waters; J. Maps; 12(5):917-35 (2016)
9. Lai, G.G., et al.; Diatoms and quality of watercourses in north-central Sardinia; Vie et Milieu – Life and Environment; 60(3):209-16 (2010)
10. Angelone, M., et al.; Fluid geochemistry of the Sardinian Rift-Campidano Graben (Sardenia, Italy): fault segmentation, seismic quiescence of geochemically "active" faults, and new constraints for selection of CO2 storage sites; Applied Geochemistry; 20:217-340 (2005)
11. Cidu, R. and Mulas, A.D.; Geochemical feature of thermal waters at Benetutti (Sardinia); Rendiconti Seminario Facolta Scienze Cagliari, 73 Fasc. 1 (2003)

12. Nahar, S., and Zhang, J.; Impact of natural water chemistry on public drinking water in Japan; Enviorn. Earth Sci.; May; 69(1):127-40 (2012)

13. Tasaki, Y., Ito, G., and Momoi, Y.; Silica urolithiasis in dogs; Kagoshima Univ. Repository; http://hdl.handle.net/10232/16977 (2013)

14. Tokuyama, A., et al.; Geochemical behavior of chemical species in the process of limestone formation. Part 1. Chemical composition of corals and limestones in the Ryukyu Islands; Geochem. J.; 6:83-92 (1972)

15. Sagae, K., et al.; Stratigraphy of the Ryukyu Group in southern Okinawa-jima, Ryuku Islands, Japan; J. of Geological Soc.; 118(2):117-136 (2012)

16. Okinawan drinking water sources; Enterprise Bureau of Okinawa; River water reservoirs 81%, River water 12%, Groundwater 6..4%; Converted seawater 0.7% (2014)

17. Iler, R.K.; The Chemistry of Silica; Wiley Interscience, New York (1979)

18. Demadis, K., et al.; Catalytic effect of magnesium ions on silicic acid polycondensation and inhibition strategies based on chelation; Industrial Eng. Chem. Research; 51:9032-40 (2012)

19. Sheikholeslami, R., et al.; Desalination and the environment water shortage – Pretreatment and the effect of cations and anions on prevention of silica fouling; Desalination; Sept.; 139(1-3):83-95 (2001)

20. Yee, N.; et al.; The effect of cyanobacteria on silica precipitation at neutral pH: implications for bacterial silicification in geothermal hot springs; Chem. Geol.; 199:83-90 (2003)

21. Tanaka, T., et al.; Silicon concentrations in maternal serum and breastmilk in the postpartum period; Nihon Eiseigaku Zasshi; Oct.; 45(4):919-25 (1990)

22. Select committee on GRAS substances – SCOGS-61, NTIS Pb 301-402/AS (1979)

23. Elefritz, R.A., Jr., et al.; AWWA Standard for Liquid Sodium Silicate; American Water Works Association; ANSI/AWWA B404-98 (1999)

24. https://en.wikipedia.org/wiki/Silicon_dioxide

25. Xie, G., et al.; Biodistribution and toxicity of intravenously administered silica nanoparticles in mice; Arch Toxicol.; 83(3):183-190 (2010)

26. Morishige, T., et al.; Suppression of nanosilica particle-induced inflammation by surface modification of the particles; Arch Toxicol.; 86(8):1297-1307 (2012)

27. Fede, C., et al.; The toxicity outcomes of silica nanoparticles (Ludox) is influenced by testing techniques and treatment modalities; Anal. Biolanal. Chem.; 404:1789-1802 (2012) –

Toxicity of silica nanoparticles on three human cell lines was 5 to 10 fold higher in serum media than non-serum media.

28. Kim, Y-R., et al.; Toxicity of colloidal silica nanoparticles administered orally for 90 days in rats; Int. J. Nanomed.; 9(Suppl. 2):67-78 (2014)

29. Coradin, T., et al.; The silicomolybdic acid spectrometric method and its application to silicate/biopolymer interaction studies; Spectroscopy; 18:567-76 (2004) – Figure 3 shows it takes 3 hours at pH 4.7 to increase OSA from 50% to 75% in a 10mM sodium silicate solution.

30. Jugdaohsingh, R., et al.; Oligomeric but not monomeric silica prevents aluminum absorption in humans; Am. J. Clin. Nutr.; 71:944-9 (2000) – Figure 2 shows it takes less than 2 weeks at pH 7.2 to increase OSA from 10% to 98% in an oligomeric silicate solution – Figure 1C shows OSA ingestion increases urinary aluminum excretion by 75% versus citrate ingestion.

31. Hadad, F.S., and Kouyoumdijiam, A.; Silica stones in humans; Urol. Int.; 41(1):70-6 (1986)

32. Katzin, W.E., et al.; Pathology of lymph nodes from patients with breast implants: a histologic and spectroscopic evaluation; Am. J. Surg. Pathol.; Apr.; 29(4):506-11 (2005)

33. Weigden, C.H. van der; Cahiers of Geochemistry – Silicon II: marine biogenic silica (2007)

34. Carmignani, L., et al.; The geological map of Sardinia (Italy) at 1:250,00 scale; J. Maps; 12(6):826-36 (2016)

35. Gursky, H.-J., and Schmidt-Effing, R.; Chapter 9 Sedimentology of radiolarities within the Nicoya Ophiolite Complex, Costa Rica, Central America; Dev. Sedimentology; 36:127-42 (1983)

36. Hem, J.D., and Roberson, C.E.; Form and stability of aluminum hydroxide complexes in dilute solution; Geological Survey Water Supply Paper 1827-A; U.S. Government Printing Office, Washington D.C. (1967)

37. Beardmore, J., et al.; What is the mechanism of formation of hydoxyaluminosilicates?; Scientific Reports; 6:30913 (2016)

38. James, B.R., et al.; An 8-hydroxyquiloline method for labile and total aluminum in soil extracts; Soil Sci. Soc. Am. J.; 47:893-97 (1983)

39. Exley, C., and Birchall, J.D.; Hydroxyaluminosilicate formation in solutions of low total aluminum concentration; Polyhedron; 11(15):1901-7 (1992)

40. Exley, C.; Reflections upon and recent insight into the mechanism of formation of hydroxyaluminosilicates and therapeutic potential of silicic acid; Coordination Chemistry Rev.; 256:82-88 (2012)

41. Wieland, E., and Stumm, E.; Dissolution kinetics of kaolinite in acidic aqueous solutions at 25°C; Geochim. Cosmochim. Acta; 56(9):3339-55 (1992)

42. Siepak, J., et al.; Speciation of aluminum released under the effect of acid rain; Polish J. Environ. Studies; 8(1):55-58 (1999)

43. Spectrum Analytics – Agronomic Library; Soil aluminum and soil test interpretation

44. Guntzer, F., et al.; Benefits of plant silicon for crops: a review; Agron. Sutain. Dev.; 32:201-13 (2012)

45. Wang, Y., et al.; Apoplastic binding of aluminum is involved in silicon-induced amelioration of aluminum toxicity in Maize; Plant Physiol.; Nov.; 136:3762-70 (2004)

46. Hammond, K.E., et al.; Aluminium/silicon interactions in barley (Hordeum vulgare L.) seedlings; Plant and Soil; 173:89-95 (1995)

47. Baylis, A.D., et al.; Effects of silicon on the toxicity of aluminium to soybean; Commun. Soil Sci. Plant Anal.; 25:537-546 (1994)

48. Galvez, L., et al.; Silicon interactions with manganese and aluminum toxicity in sorghum; J. Plant Nutr.; 10:1139-47 (1987)

49. Jones, D.L., et al.; Spatial coordination of aluminum uptake, production of reactive oxygen species, callose production and wall rigidification in maize roots; Plant Cell. Environ.; 29:1309-18 (2006)

50. Law, C., and Exley, C.; New insight into silica deposition in horsetail (*Equisetum arvense*); BMC Plant Biol.; 11:112 1-9 (2011)

51. Ryder, M., et al.; The use of root growth and modelling data to investigate amelioration of aluminum toxicity by silicon in *Picea abies* seedlings; J. Inorg. Biochem.; Sept., 97:52-58 (2003)

52. Cocker, K.M., et al.; The amelioration of aluminum toxicity by silicon in higher plants: Solution chemistry or an in planta mechanism?; Physiologia Plantarum; 104(4):608-14 (1998)

53. Zuo, X. et al.; Dating rice remains through phytolith carbon-14 study reveals domestication at the beginning of the Halocene; PNAS; May; 317260327 (2017)

54. Massot, N., et al.; Callose production as an indicator of aluminum toxicity in bean cultivars; J. Plant Nutrition; 22(1):1-10 (2008)

55. Vessala, T., at al.; Effect of leaf water potential on internal humidity and CO_2 dissolution: Reverse transpiration and improved water use efficiency under negative pressure; Frontiers in Plant Sci.; Feb.; 8:54 1-10 (2017)

56. Burkhardt, J.; Hygroscopic particles on leaves: nutrient or desiccants?; Ecological Monographs; 80(3):369-99 (2010)

57. Apostolakos, P., et al.; The role of callose in guard-cell wall differentiation and stomatal pore formation in the fern *Asplenium nidus*; Annuals of Botany; 104:1373-87 (2009)

58. Carnelli, A.L., et al.; Aluminum in the opal silica reticule of phytoliths: A new tool in palaeoecological studies; Am. J. of Botany; 89(2):346-51 (2002)

59. Birchall, J.D., et al.; Acute toxicity of aluminum to fish eliminated in silicon-rich waters; Nature; 338:146-48 (1989)

60. Exley, C., et al.; Hydroxyaluminosilicates and acute aluminum toxicity in fish; J.Theoretical Biol.; 189(2):133-39 (1997)

61. Desouky, M., et al.; Aluminum-dependent regulation of intracellular silicon in the aquatic invertebrate *Lymnaea stagnalis*; PNAS; March 99:3394-99 (2002)

62. Carlisle, E.M., and Curran, M.J.; Effect of dietary silicon and aluminum on silicon and aluminum levels in rat brain; Alzheimer Dis. Assoc. Disord.; 1(2):83-9 (1987)

63. Domingo, L., et al.; Age related effects of aluminum ingestion on brain aluminum accumulation and behavior in rats; Life Sci.; 58(17):1387-95 (1996)

64. Belles, M., et al.; Silicon reduces aluminum accumulation in rats: Relevance to the aluminum hypothesis of Alzheimer's disease; Alzheimer Disease Associated Disorders; 12(2):83-87 (1998)

65. Mold, M., et al.; Aluminum in brain tissue in autism; J. Trace Elements in Med. Biol.; March; 46:76-82 (2018)

66. Sundreman, F.W. Jr.; Nasal toxicity, carcinogenicity, and olfactory uptake of metals; Annals Clin. Lab. Sci.; 31(1):3-24(2001)

67. Zatta, P., et al.; Deposition of aluminum in brain tissues of rats exposed to inhalation of aluminum acetylacetonate; Neuroreport; Sept.; 4(9):119-22 (1993)

68. Perl, D.P. and Good, P.F.; Uptake of aluminum into central nervous system along nasal-olfactory pathways; Lancet; May; 1(8540:1028 (1987)

69. Divine, K.K., et al.; Quantitative particle-induced x-ray emission imaging of rat olfactory epithelium applied to the permeability of rat epithelium to inhaled aluminum; Chem. Res. Toxicol.; 12(7):575-81 (1999)

70. Drueke, T.D.; Intestinal absorption of aluminum in renal failure; Nephrol. Dial. Transplant; 17[Suppl. 2]:13-16 (2002)

71. Reffitt, D.M., et al.; Silicic acid: its gastrointestinal uptake and urinary excretion in man and effects on aluminum excretion; J. Inorg. Biochem.; 76:141-47 (1999)

72. Carlisle, E.M.; Silicon as an essential trace element in animal nutrition; Silicon Biochemistry; Ciba Foundation Symposium 121; John Wiley & Sons (1986)

73. Davenward, S., et al.; Silicon-rich mineral water as a non-invasive test of the 'aluminum hypothesis' in Alzheimer's disease; J. Alzheimer's Dis.; 33(2):423-30 (2013)

74. Minshal, C., et al.; Aluminum in human sweat; J. Trace elem. Med. Biol.; 28:87-88 (2014)

75. Exley, C.; Aluminum toxicity: a major threat to brain health; Alzheimer's and Dementia Summit; Hosted by J. Landsman; July 31 (2016)

76. https://en.wikipedia.org/wiki/Aluminium-26

77. Edwardson, J.A., et al.; Effect of silicon on gastrointestinal absorption of aluminum; The Lancet; 342(8865):211-12 (1993)

78. Exley, C., et al.; Non-invasive therapy to reduce the body burden of aluminum in Alzheimer's disease; J. Alzheimer's Disease; 10:17-24 (2006)

79. Sripanyakorn, S., et al.; The comparative absorption of silicon from different foods and food supplements; Br. J. Nutr.; Sept.; 102(6):825-34 (2009)

80. Bellia, J.P., Birchall, J.D., and Roberts, N.B.; The role of silicic acid in the renal excretion of aluminum; Ann. Clin. Lab. Sci.; June, 26(3):227-33 (1996)

81. Adler, A.J. and Berlyne, G.M.; Duodenal aluminum absorption in the rat: effect of vitamin D; Gastrintest. Liner Physiol.; 12:G209-G213 (1985)

82. Dressman, J.B., et al.; Upper gastrointestinal (GI) pH in young, health, men and women; Pharma. Res.; 7(7):756-61 (1990)

83. Manz, F.; et al.; Water balance throughout the adult life span in a German population; British J. Nutri.; 107:1673-1681

84. Gagnon, D. and Kenny, G.P.; Sex differences in thermoeffector responses during exercise at fixed requirements for heat loss; J. Appl. Physiol.; Sept.; 113(5):746-57 (1985)

85. Van Dyke, K., et al.; Indications of silicon essentiality in humans – Serum concentrations in Belgian children and adults, including pregnant women; Biological Trace Element Res.; 77:25-32 (2000)

86. Jugdaohsingh, R.; Silicon and bone health; J. Nutr. Health Aging: 11(2):99-110 (2007)

87. Jugdaohsingh, R., et al.; Dietary silicon is positively associated with bone mineral density in men and postmenopausal women; J. Bone Mineral Res.; 19(2):297-307 (2004)

88. Reffitt, D.M., et al.; Orthosilicic acid stimulates collagen type I synthesis and osteoblastic differentiation in human osteoblast-like cells in vitro; Bone; Feb.; 32(2):127-135 (2003)

89. Guinness Book of World Recdords; London, U,K.; Guinness; 67 (2007)

90. Robine, J.M. and Saito, Y.; Survival beyond age 100: the case of Japan; Popul. Dev. Rev.; 29:208-28 (2003)

91. Willcox, D.C., et al.; They really are that old: A validation study of centenarian prevalence in Okinawa; J. Gerontology:Biol. Sci.; 63A(4):338-49 (2008)

92. Japan Ministry of Health, Labor and Welfare (2006)

93. Kugel; Population Census of Japan, National Institute of Population and Social Security Research (2010)

https://upload.wikimedia.org/wikipedia/commons/7/76/Population_of_Okinawa_prefecture%2C_Japan.png

94. Wilcox, D.C., et al.; Caloric restriction and human longevity: what can we learn from the Okinawans?; Biogeronotolgy; 7:173-77 (2006)

95. Takata, H., et al.; Influence of major histocompatibility complex region genes on human longevity among Okinawan-Japanese centenarians and nonagenarians; Lancet; 2:824-6 (1987)

96. Bernstein, A.M., et al.; First autopsy study of an Okinawan centariean: Absence of many age-related diseases; J. Gerontology: Medical Sciences; 59A(11):1195-99 (2004)

97. Lie, J.T., and Hammond, P.I.; Pathology of the senescent heart: anatomic observations on 237 autopsy studies of patients 90-105 years old; Mayo Clinic Proc.; 63:552-64 (1988)

98. Roberts, W.C.; The heart at necroscopy in centenarians; Am. J. Cardiol.; 81:1224-25 (1998)

99. Alfthan, G., et al.; Plasma homocysteine and cardiovascular disease mortality; Lancet; Feb.; 349(9049):397 (1997)

100.   Waly, M. et al.; Activation of methionine synthase by insulin-like growth factor-1 and dopamine: a target for neurodevelopmental toxins and thimerosal; Mol. Psychiatry; 9:348-70 (2004)

101.   Waly, M.I-A. and Deth, R.; Neurodevelopmental toxins deplete glutathione and inhibit folate and vitamin B12-dependent methionine synthase activity – a link between oxidative stress and autism; FASEB J.; 22:894-1 (2008)

102.   Ogura, C., et al.; Prevalence of senile dementia in Okinawa, Japan; Int. J. Epidemiol.; 24:373-80 (1995)

103.   Yamada, M., et al.; Prevalence and risks of dementia in the Japanese population: RERF's adult health study Hiroshima subjects; J. Am. Geriatr. Soc.; 47:189-95 (1999)

104.   AD Death Rate Data 2016 worldlifeexpectancy.com/cause-of-death/alzheimers-dementia/by-country/

105.   World Health Organization; Hormone-Dependent Cancer Risk (1996)

106.   Japan Ministry of Health and Welfare; Hormone-Dependent Cancer Risk (1996)

107.   Prakash, R., et al.; Homologous recombination and human health roles of BRCA1, BRCA2, and associated proteins; Cold Spring Harbor Perspectives in Biology; April; 7(4):a016600 (2015)

108.   Wilson, C.A., et al.; Localization of human BRCA1 and its loss in high-grade, non-inherited breast carcinomas; Nat. Genet.; 21(2):236-40 (1999)

109.   Jacinto, F.V., and Esteller, M.; Mutator pathways unleased by epigenetic silencing in human cancer; Mutagenesis; 22(4):247-53 (2007)

110.   Farasani, A., and Darbre P.D.; Effects of aluminum chloride and aluminum chlorohydrate on DNA repair in MCF-10A immortalized non-transformed human breast epithelial cells; J. Inorg. Biochem.; Nov.; 152:186-9 (2015)

111.   Rosen, E.M., Fan, S., Goldberg, I.D.; BRCA1 and prostate cancer; Cancer Invest.; 19(4):396-412 (2001)

112.   Toyama, E.; Limnology studies on Fukuji Reservoir at Higashi-son, Okinawa Island - Part 1. Physiochemical factors and plankton; Jap. J. Limnol. 43(4):246-53 (1982)

113.   Ross, P.D., et al.; A comparison of hip fracture incidents among Native Japanese, Japanese Americans, and American Caucsians; April; Am. J. Epidemiol.; 133(8):801-9 (1991)

114.   Suzuki, M., et al.; Japanese J. Bone Res.; 63:166-72 (1995)

115.   Rico, H., et al.; Effect of silicon supplements on osteopenia induced by ovariectomy in rats; Calcif. Tissue Int.; 66(1):53-5 (2000)

116.   Bae, Y.J., et al.; Short-term administration of water-soluble silicon improves mineral density of femur and tibia in ovariectomized rats; Biol. Trace Elem. Res.; 124(2):157-63 (2008)

117.   Kim, M.H., et al.; Silicon supplementation improves bone mineral density of calcium-deficient ovariectomized rats by reducing bone resorption; Biol. Trace Elem. Res.; 128(3):239-47 (2009)

118.   Rondeau, V., et al.; Aluminum and silica in drinking water and the risk of Alzheimer's disease or cognitive decline; findings from 15-year follow-up of the PAQUID cohort; Am. J. Epidemiol.; 169:489-96 (2009)

119.   Deiana, L., et al.; The Sardinian study of extreme longevity; Aging Clin. Exp. Res.; 11:142-149 (1999)

120.   Poulain, M., et al.; Identification of a geographic area characterized by extreme longevity in the Sardinia Island: The AKEA Study; Experimental Gerontology; 39(9):1423-29 (2004)

121.   Poulain, M., et al.; A population where men live as long as women: Villagrande Strisaili, Sardinia; J. Aging Res.; Article ID 153756 (2011)

122.   Padedda, B.M.; IT10 – Lake ecosystems of Sardinia; LTER_EU_IT_010 (2006)

123.   De Waele, J.; The hydrogeological rebus of the coastal karst of Orosei (East Sardina, Italy; Proceedings of the 14th Internat. Cong. Speleology, Athens-Kalamos;21-28 Aug. (2005)

124.   Lai, G.G. et al.; Epilithic diatom assemblages and environmental quality of the Su Gologone karst sprig (central-eastern Sardinia, Italy; Acta. Bot. Croat.; 75(1):129-43 (2016)

125.   Sanna, F., et al.; Development of a sustainable water management for the Su Gologone karst spring (Sardinia, Italy); 3rd National Meeting on Hydrology; Cagiari, 14-16 June (2017)

126.   Harper, H.E., and Knoll, A.H.; Silica, diatoms, and Cenozoic radiolarian evolution; Geology; 3:175-177 (1975)

127.   Maldonado, M., et al.; Decline in Mesozoic reef-building sponges explained by silicon limitation; Nature; Oct.; 401:785-88 (1999)

128.   Halliday, A.K., et al.; Sex and gender differences in autistic spectrum disorder: summarizing evidence gaps and identifying emerging areas of priority; Mol. Autism; 6:36 (2015)

129.   D'Eufemia, P., et al.; Abnormal intestinal permeability in children with autism; Acta Paeditr.; Sep.; 85(9):1079-91 (1996)

130.   Blaurock-Busch, E., et al.; Toxic metals and essential elements in hair and severity of symptoms among children with autism; Maedica, J. Clin. Med.; 7(1):30-48 (2012)

131.   Mohamed, F.E.B., et al.; Assessment of hair aluminum, lead, and mercury in a sample of autistic Egyptian children: Environmental risk factors of heavy metals in autism; Behavioral Neurology; Article ID 545674:1-9 (2015)

132.   Mold, M., et al.; Aluminum in brain tissue in autism; J. Trace Elements in Med. Biol.; Manuscript 1-23 (2017)

133.   Panagiotakos, D.B., et al.; Sociodemographic and lifestyle statistics of oldest old people (>80 years) living in Ikaria Island: The Ikaria Study; Cardiology Res. Practice; Article ID 679187 (2011)

134.   Poulain, M. and Pes, G.M.; Report on the validation of the exceptional longevity in Ikaria; Unpublished Internal Report; National Geographic (2009)

135.   Stefanadis, C.I.; Unveiling the secrets of longevity: The Ikaria Study; Hellenic J. Cardiol.; 52:479-480 (2011)

136.   Schwarz, K., et al.; Inverse relation of silicon in drinking water and atherosclerosis in Finland; Lancet; Mar.; 1(8010):538-39 (1977)

137.   At the heart of Ikaria; Does a Greek island harbor the secret to longevity? CardioVascular Institute at Beth Israel Deaconess Medical Center (2016)

138.   Tsagarakis, K.P., et al.; County report Greece, Aqualibrium, European water management between regulation and competition, (2002) – Available at http://www.oieau.fr/aqualibrium/Aqualibrium_08.pdf

139.   European Academics Science Advisory Council; Groundwater in the southern member states of the European Union: an assessment of current knowledge and future prospects; County Report for Greece

140.   Karavoltsos, S., et al.; Evaluation of the quality of drinking water in regions of Greece; Desalination; 224:317-29 (2008)

141.   Bellos, D., et al.; Nutrient chemistry of river Pinios (Thessalia, Greece); Environ. Int.; 30:105-15 (2004)

142.   Ludwig, W., et al.; River discharges of water and nutrients to the Mediterranean and Black Sea: Major drivers for ecosystem changes during the past and future decades?; Progress in Oceanography; 80:199-217 (2009)

143.   Margat, J., and Treyer, S.; L'eau des Mediterraneens: situation et perspectives, Map Technical Report Series No. 158, 366 pp (2004) (Available from http://www.unepmap.org/)

144.   Stamatis, G., and Gartzos, E.; The silica supersaturated waters of northern Evia and eastern central Greece; Hydrol. Process.; 13:2833-45 (1999)

145.   Baumgartner, P. and Bernouli, D. Stratigraphy and radiolarian fauna in a Late Jurassic-Early Cretaceous section near Achladi, Evia, Eastern Greece, Eclogaae Geol. Helv., 69, 601-26 (1976)

146.   Rosero-Bixby, L., et al.; The Nicoya Region of Costa Rica: A high longevity island for elderly males; Vienna Yearbook of Population Research; 11:109-36 (2013)

147.   Rosero-Bixby, L., and Dow, W.; Predicting mortality with biomarkers: A population-based prospective cohort study for Elderly Costa Ricans; Population Health Metrics; 10(11):1-15 (2012)

148.   Castrillo, W.V.; Gunanacaste will start drinking water from reservoirs in 2018; June 23; 13:48 (2016)

149.   Rosero-Bixby, L., The exceptional high life expectancy of Costa Rica Nonagenarians; Cenus 61(1):673-691 (2008)

150.   Hannah, R.S., et al.; Origin of silicic volcanic rocks in Central Costa Rica: a study of a chemically variable ash-flow sheet in the Tiribi Tuff; Bull. Volcanol.; 64:117-33 (2002)

151.   Calvo, C.; Provenance of plutonic detritus in cover sandstones of Nicoya Complex, Costa Rica: Cretaceous unroofing history of a Mesozoic ophiolite sequence; GSA Bulletin; 115(7):832-844 (2003)

152.   Gursky, H.-J., and Schmidt-Effing, R.; Sedimentology of radiolarites within the Nicoya Ophiolite Complex, Costa Rica, Central America; Dev. Sedimentology; 36:127-42 (1983)

153.   Bandini, A.N., et al.; Late Cretaceous and Paleogene Radiolaria from the Nicoya Peninsula, Costa Rica: a tectonostratigraphic application; Stratigraphy; 5(1):3-21 (2008)

154.   Michels, A.; Effects of sewage water on diatom (Bacillariophyceae) and water quality in two tropical streams in Costa Rica; Rev. Biol. Trop.; 46 Suppl. 6; 153-175 (1998)

155.   Las Cruces Biological Station Brochure "… Java River the source of water to the town of San Vito for many years."

156.   https://bluezones.com/exploration/loma-linda-california/

157.   Spector, N.; What 'blue z' city Loma Linda, California can teach us about living longer; NBCNews.com; Better by Today; April (2019)

158.   Leaf, A.; Long-lived populations: extreme old age; J. Am. Geriatr. Soc.; 30:485-87 (1982)

159.   Krach, C.A., and Velkoff, V.A.; Bureau of the Census, Current Population Reports; Series P23-199RV; Centenarians in the United States; Washington, DC; U.S. Government Printing Office (1999)

160.   Beeson, W.L., et al.; Chronic disease among Seventh-day Adventists; Cancer; 64:591-97 (1989)

161.   Fraser, G.E., et al.; Ten years of life – is it a matter of choice; Arch Intern. Med.; July; 161:1645-52 (2001)

162.   Chan, J.; et al.; Water, other fluids, and fatal coronary heart disease: The Adventists Study; Am. J. Epidem.; 155(9): 827-33 (2002)

163.   Bleich, S., et al.; Moderate alcohol consumption in social drinkers raises plasma homocysteine levels – a contradiction of the French Paradox?; Alcohol Alcoholism; 36(3):189-92 (2001)

164.   International longevity comparisons; Stat. Bull. Metrop. Insur. Co.; 73:10-15 (1992)

165.   Xiao, Y., et al.; Dietary protein and plasma total homocysteine, cysteine, concentrations in coronary angiographic subjects; Nutr. J.; 12:144-54 (2013)

166.   Fraser, G.E.; Associations between diet and cancer, ischemic heart disease, and all-cause mortality in non-Hispanic white California Seventh-day Adventists; Am. J. Clin. Nutr.; 70(suppl.):532S-8S (1999)

167.   Sopik, V., et al.; BRCA1 and BRCA2 mutations and the risk for colorectal cancer; Clin. Genet.; May; 87(5):411-8 (2015)

168. Paffenbarger, R.S., et al.; Physical activity, all-cause mortality, and longevity of college alumini; N. Engl. J. Med.; 314:605-13 (1986)

169. Pekkanen, J., et al.; Reduction of premature mortality by high physical activity: a 20-year follow-up of middle-aged Finnish men; Lancet; 1:1473-77 (1987)

170. Fraser, G.E., and Shavlik, D.; Risk factors, lifetime risk, and age at onset of breast cancer; Ann. Epidemiol.; Aug.; 7(6):375-82 (1997)

171. City of Loma Linda - Annual water quality report (2015)

172. Horick, P.J., and Steinhilber, W.J.; Jordan Aquifer of Iowa - Miscellaneous Map Series 6 (1978)

173. Siegle, D.I.; Geochemistry of the Cambrian-Ordovician Aquifer System in the Northern Midwest, United States, Regional Aquifer-System Analysis; U.S. Geological Survey Professional Paper 1405D (1989)

174. Crouse, D.N.; Unreported laboratory results (2015)

175. Whittier, J.; The value of tap water: A comparison of bottled, filtered, and tap water using the MWRA as a case study; Environ. Management I Harvard Extension School; Dec. 19 (2007)

176. Giem, P., et al.; The incidence of dementia and intake of animal products: preliminary findings from the Adventist Health Study; Neuroepidemiology; 12(1):28-36 (1993)

177. Joshipura, K.J., et al.; Fruit and vegetable intake in relation to risk of ischemic stroke; JAMA; Oct.; 282(13):1233-39 (1999)

178. Joshipura, K.J., et al.; The effect of fruit and vegetable intake on risk for coronary heart disease; Annals Int. Med.; 134(12):1106-14 (2001)

179. D'Imperio, M., et al.; Silicon biofortification of leafy vegetables and its bioaccessibility in edible plants; J. Sci. Food Agri.; 96(3):751-56 (2016)

180. Wang, M., et al.; Effect of silicon application on silicon content in "Fugi" apples in Loess Plateau; Comm. Soil Sci. Plant Anal.; 47(20):2325-33 (2016)

181. Henriet, C., et al.; Effects, distribution, and uptake of silicon in banana (*Nusa app.*) under controlled conditions; Plant and Soil; 287:359-74 (2006)

182. Zhang, N., et al.; Applying silicate fertilizer increases both yield and quality of table grape (Vitis vinifera L.) grown on calceous grey soil; Scientia Horticulturae; Nov.; 225:757-63 (2017)

183.   Blaich, R. and Grundhofer, H.; Uptake of silica by grapevines from soil and recirculating nutrient solution; Vitis; 36(4):161-66 (1997)

184.   Bartoli, F., and Wilding, L.P.; Dissolution of biogenic opal as a function of its physical and chemical properties; Soil Sci. Soc. Am. J.; 44(4):873-78 (1980)

185.   Ma, J.F., and Takahashi, E.; Soil, fertilizer, and plant silicon research in Japan; Elsevier, Amsterdam; (2002)

186.   Davis, D.R.; Declining fruit and vegetable nutrient composition: What is the evidence?; HortScience; Feb.; 44(1):15-19 (2009)

187.   Guntzer, F., et al.; Benefits of plant silicon for crops: a review; Agron. Substain. Dev.; 32:201-13 (2012)

188.   Tubana, B.S., et al.; A review of silicon in soils and plants and its role in US agriculture: History and future perspectives; Soil Sci.; 181:393-411 (2016)

189.   Bernal, J.; Response of rice and sugarcane to magnesium silicate in different soils of Columbia South America; Paper presented at the IV Silicon in Agriculture Conference, Brazil; Carrera 57 #14-44, Bogata, Columbia (2008)

190.   Kaufmann, K.; Silica: The Forgotten Nutrient; Alive Books (1993)

191.   Sripanyakorn, S., et al.; The silicon content of beer and its bioavailability in healthy volunteers; British J. Nutrition; 91:403-409 (2004)

192.   Jugdaohsingh, R., et al.; Dietary silicon intake and absorption; Am. J. Clin. Nutri.; 75(5):887-93 (2002)

193.   Powell, J.J., et al.; A provisional database for silicon content of foods in the United Kingdom; British J. of Nutrition; 94:804-812 (2005)

194.   Taylor, G.A., et al.; Gastrointestinal absorption of aluminum in Alzheimer's disease: Response to aluminum citrate; Age Ageing; Mar.; 21(2):81-90 (1992)

195.   Shimizu, H., et al.; A correlative study of the aluminum content and aging changes of the brain in non-elderly subjects; Nihon Ronen Igakkai Zasshi; Dec.; 31(12)950-60 (1994)

196.   Rao, V.; World's oldest family says this breakfast staple is the key to a long life; Today.com Aug. 1 (2017)

197.   McNeill, M.; The Scots kitchen: Its traditions and recipes; (1929)

198.   Sutherland, C.; Blog Post: Sowans – the fermented oat food; Past and Pottage – Food history for the present; Includes modern recipe for sowans; Jan 30 (2017)

199.   Barclay, E.; Eating to break 100: Longevity diet tips from the blue zs; NPR April (2015)

200.   Todoriki, H., et al.; The effects of post-war dietary change on longevity and health in Okinawa; Okinawan J. Am. Studies; 52-61 (2004)

201.   Kagawa, Y.; Impact of westernization on the nutrition of Japanese: Changes in physique, cancer, longevity, and centenarians; Preventative Med.; June; 205-217 (1978)

202.   Crago, S.; Born in the USA, eaten in Okinawa; The Japan Times; Oct. 23 (2015)

203.   Onishi, N.; On U.S. fast food more Okinawans grow super-sized; Urasoe Journal; March 30 (2004)

204.   Pes G.M., et al.; Lifestyle and nutrition related to male longevity in Sardinia: An ecological study; Nutr. Metab. Cardiovascular Disease; March, 212-19 (2013)

205.   Fermi. C.; Decadenza, risanamento e spesa; Tipografia; vol. 1-3; Regioni malariche, Sardegna (1934)

206.   Peretti, G.; Rapporti tra alimentazione e caratteri antropometrici; Studio statistico-biometrico in Sardegna; Quaderni Della Nutrizione; IX:69-130 (1943)

207.   Wagner, P.L., and Mikesell, W.; Readings in cultural geography; Chicago; Univ. of Chicago Press (1962)

208.   Institute of Nutrition of Central America and Panama (INCAP) and the Interdepartmental Committee on Nutrition for National Development (ICNND); Tables 3, 4, and 106 in Nutritional Evaluation of the Population of Central America and Panama (1965-67)

209.   Sidhu, S.K. and Nicholson, J.W.; A review of glass-ionomer cements for clinical dentistry; J. Funct. Biomater.; 7(3):16 (2016)

210.   Hantson, P., et al.; Fatal encephalopathy after otoneurosurgery procedure with an aluminum containing biomaterial; J. Toxicol. Clin. Toxicol.; 33(6):645-8 (1995)

211.   Alfrey, A.C.; Aluminum toxicity in patients with chronic renal failure; Ther. Drug Monit.; 15(6):593-97 (1993)

212.   House, R.A.; Factors affecting plasma aluminum concentrations in nonexposed workers; J. Occup. Med.; 34:1013-17 (1992)

213.   Liao, Y.H., et al.; Biological monitoring of exposure to aluminum, gallium, indium, arsenic, and antimony in optoelectronic workers; J. Occup. Environ. Med.; 46(9):931-36 (2004)

214.   Banks, W.A., and Kastin, A.J.; Aluminum alters the permeability of the blood-brain barrier to some non-peptides; Neuropharmacology; may; 24(5):407-12 (1985)

215.   Kaya, M., et al.; Effect of aluminum on the blood-brain barrier permeability during nitric oxide-blockade-induced chronic hypertension in rats; Biol. Trace Elem. Res.; Jun.; 92(3):221-30 (2003)

216.   Song, Y., et al.; Effects of acute exposure to aluminum on blood-brain barrier and the protection of zinc; Neurosci. Lett.; Nov.; 445(1):42-6 (2008)

217.   Chen, Li., et al.; Manufactured aluminum oxide nanoparticles decrease expression of tight junction proteins in brain vasculature; J. Neuroimmune Pharmacol.; 3(4):286-95 (2008)

218.   Chadobski, A., et al.; Blood-brain barrier pathophysiology in traumatic brain injury; Transl. Stroke Res.; Dec.; 2(4):492-516 (2011)

219.   Pogue, A.I., et al.; Metal-sulfate induced generation of ROS in human brain cells: detection using an isomeric mixture of 5- and 6-carboxy-2',7'-dichlorofluoresein diacetate (carboxy-DCFDA) as a cell permeant tracer, Int. J. Mol.; 13:9615-26 (2012)

220.   Mooradian, A.D.; Effect of aging on the blood-brain barrier; Neurobiology of Aging; 9:31-9 (1988)

221.   Kaya, M., et al.; Effect of aluminum on the blood-brain barrier permeability during nitric oxide-blockade-induced chronic hypertension in rats; Biol. Trace Elem. Res.; Jun.; 92(3):221-30 (2003)

222.   Farrall, A.J. and Wardlaw, J.M.; Blood-brain barrier: ageing and microvascular disease - - systematic review and meta-analysis; Neurobiol. Aging; Mar.; 30(3):337-52 (2009)

223.   Kortekaas, R., et al.; Blood-brain barrier dysfunction in parkinsonian midbrain in vivo; Ann. Neurol.; 57:176-9 (2005)

224.   Gray, M.T. and Woulf, J.M.; Striatal blood-brain barrier permeability in Parkinson's disease; J. Cerebral Blood Flow and Metab.; 35:747-50 (2015)

225.   Garcia-Monoco, J.C., et al.; Adherence of the Lyme disease spirochete to glial cells and cells of glial origin; J. Infectious Dis.; Oct. 160(3):497-506 (1989)

226.   Alzheimer, A.; Uber eine eigenartige erkrankung der hirnrinde; Zentralbl Nervenheit Psychiatr; 30, 177179 (1907)

227.   Das, S.K., and Yin, W.; The worldwide aluminum economy: The current state of the industry; JOM; Nov,; 59(11):57-63 (2007) Aluminum production 1986-2006 Primary Worldwide Aluminum Production: 0.18mt in 1918, 2.0mt in 1952, 32.0mt in 2005

228.   Brown, S.C.; Minerals in the World Economy; Minerals Year Book; 1-44 (1968) Table 5 World Production of Aluminum: 4.53mt in1960

229.   World Aluminum – Primary Aluminum Production - http://www.world-aluminium.org/statistics/primary-aluminium-production/ 12.0mt in 1973, 12.3mt in 1975, 15.4mt in 1980, 15.5mt in 1985, 19.5mt in 1990, 19.6mt in 1995, 24.7mt in 2000, 31.9mt in 2005 42.3mt in 2010, 53.9mt in 2014

230.   Katzman, R.; et al.; Alzheimer's disease: senile dementia and related disorders; New York; Raven Press (1978) Number of People with Alzheimer's in U.S.: 1.2 million in 1976

231.   U.S. General Accounting Office; Alzheimer's disease; Estimates of prevalence in the U.S. (1998) Number of People with Alzheimer's in U.S.: 1.9 million in 1995

232.   Plassman, B.L., et al.; Prevalence of dementia in the United States: The aging, demographics, and memory study; Neuroepidemiology; 29:125-32 (2007) Number of People with Alzheimer's in U.S.: 2.4 million in 2002

233.   U.S. Alzheimer's Association; Alzheimer's disease facts and figures (2016) Number of People with Alzheimer's in U.S.: 5.4 million in 2016

234.   Lotter, V.; Epidemiology of autistic conditions in young children; Social Psychiatry; 1(3):124-35 (1966) Autism rate for children born in 1960 1/2500

235.   Hertz-Picciotto, I., and Delwiche, L.; The rise of autism rate and the role of age at diagnosis; Epidemiology; 20(1):84-90 (2009) Autism rate for Californian children born from 1985 to 1996 rose 60%. Birth year and autism rates based upon a 60% rise every decade: 1980 1/200, 1990 1/150, 2000 1/88

236.   CDC Autism Data - Birth year and autism rates: 1992 1/150, 2002 1/88, 2016 1/36

237.   CDC U.S. Annual births all races by year: 1960 4.26 million, 1980 3.61 million, 2000 4.06 million, 2016 3.95 million

238.   McLachlan, D.R.C., et al.; Risk for neuropathologically confirmed Alzheimer's disease and residual aluminum in municipal drinking water employing weighted residential histories; Neurology; 46:401-5 (1996)

239.   Martyn, C.N., et al.; Geographic relation between Alzheimer's disease and aluminum in drinking water; Lancet; 1:59-62 (1989)

240.   Flaten, T.P.; Geographical associations between aluminum in drinking water and death rates with dementia (including Alzheimer's disease), Parkinson's disease, and amyotrophic lateral sclerosis inn Norway; Environ. Geochem. Health; 12:152-67 (1990)

241.   Neri, L.C., and Hewitt, D.; Aluminum, Alzherimer's disease, and drinking water; Lancet; 338:390 (1991)

242.   Flaten, T.P.; An investigation of the chemical composition of Norwegian drinking water and its possible relationships with the epidemiology of some diseases. Dept. of Chem.; Norwegian Univ. Sci. and Tech., Trondheim, Norway (1986)

243.   Vogt, T.; Water quality and health: Study of a possible relation between aluminum in drinking water and dementia. Sosiale og Okonomiske Studier no. 61. Oslo: Statistics Norway (1986)

244.   Forbes, W.F., et al.; Geochemical risk factors for mental functioning, based upon the Ontario Longitudinal Study of Aging (LSA) V. Comparison of the results, relevant to aluminum water concentrations, obtained from LSA and death certificates mentioning dementia; Can. J. Aging; 14:642-56 (1995)

245.   Canadian Study of Health and Aging Group; The incidence of dementia in Canada in 1991; Neurology; July; 55(1):66-73 (2000)

246.   Rondeau, V., et al.; Aluminum and silica in drinking water and the risk of Alzheimer's disease or cognitive decline: findings from 15-year follow-up of the PAQUID cohort, Am. J. Epidemiol. 169:489-96 (2009)

247.   Rondeau, V., et al.; Relation between aluminum concentrations in drinking water and Alzheimer's disease: an 8-year follow-up study; Am. J. Epidemiol. 152:59-66 (2000)

248.   Gillette-Guyonnet, S., et al.; Cognitive impairment and composition of drinking water in women: findings of the EPIDOS study; Am. J. Clin. Nutr.; 81:897-902 (2005)

249.   Ward, A., et al.; Prevalence of apolipoprotein E4 genotype and homozygotes (APOE e4/4) among patients diagnosed with Alzheimer's disease: A systematic review and meta-analysis; Neuroepidemiology; 38:1-17 (2012)

250.   Chen, Y., et al.; Low prevalence and clinical effect of vascular risk factors in early-onset Alzheimer's disease; J. Alzheimer's Dis.; 60:1045-54 (2017)

251.   Bird, T.D.; Early-onset familial Alzheimer disease; GeneReviews [Internet]; Natl. Cntr. Biotech. Info., U.S. Nat. Lib. Med.; Oct. (2012)

252.   Exley, C., and Vickers, T.; Elevated brain aluminum and early onset Alzheimer's disease in an individual occupationally exposed to aluminum: a case report; J. Med. Case Reports; 8:41 (2014)

253.   Crapper, D.R., Krishnan, S.S., Dalton, A.J.; Brain aluminum distribution in Alzheimer's disease and experimental neurofibrillary degeneration; Science, May, 180(4085):511-3 (1973)

254.   Virk, S.A. and Eslick, G.D.; Aluminum levels in brain, serum, and cerebrospinal fluid are higher in Alzheimer's disease cases than in controls: A series of meta-analyses; J. Alzheimers Dis.; 47(3):629-38 (2015)

255.   Skillback, T., et al.; Cerebrospinal fluid tau and amyloid-β1-42 in patients with dementia; Brain; Sept.; 138(Pt 9):2716-31 (2015)

256.   Kanai, M., et al.; Longitudinal study of cerebrospinal fluid levels of tau, AB1-40 and AB 1-42(43) in Alzheimer's disease: A study in Japan; Annals of Neurology; 44(1):17-20 (1998)

257.   Maruyama, M., et al.; Imaging of tau pathology in a tauopathy mouse model and in Alzheimer patients compared to normal controls; Neruon; Sept.; 79:1094-1108 (2013)

258.   Higuchi, M., et al.; 19F and 1H MRI detection of amyloid beta plaque in vivo; Nat. Neurosci.; Apr.; 8(4):527-33 (2005)

259.   Lu, Z-Y, et al.; Aluminum chloride induces retinal changes in the rat; Toxicol. Sci.; 66:253-60 (2002)

260.   Pogue, A.I., et al.; Progressive inflammatory pathology in the retina of aluminum-fed 5xFAD transgenic mice; J. Inorg. Biochem.; Nov.; 152:206-0 (2015)

261.   Jentsch, A., et al.; Retinal fluorescence lifetime imaging ophthalmoscopy measures depend on the severity of Alzheimer's disease; Acta Ophthalmologica; 93: e241-47 (2015)

262.   Koronyo, Y., et al.; Retinal amyloid pathology and proof-of-concept imaging trial in Alzheimer's disease; Aug,; JCL Insight; 2(16); (2017)

263.   Negash, S., et al.; Resilient brain aging: Characterization of discordance between Alzheimer's disease pathology and cognition; Curr. Alzheimer Res.; 10(8):844-51 (2013)

264.   White, C.C.; et al.; Identification of genes associated with dissociation of cognitive performance and neuropathological burden: Multistep analysis of genetic, epigenetic, and

transcriptional data; PLOS Med.; 14(4):e1002287 (2017) – see Table 1. Demographic characteristics of participants

265.   Mirza, A., et al.; Aluminum in brain tissue in familial Alzheimer's disease; J. Trace Elements in Medicine and Biology; Mar.; 40:30-36 (2017)

266.   Andrasi, E., et al.; Brain Al, Mg, and P contents of control and Alzheimer-diseased patients; J. Alzheimer's Dis.; 7:273-84 (2005)

267.   Rusina, R., et al.; Higher aluminum concentrations in Alzheimer's disease after Box-Cox data transformation; Neurotox. Res.; 20, 329-33 (2011)

268.   Xu, N., et al.; Brain aluminum in Alzheimer's disease using an improved GFAAS method; Neurotoxicology; 13:735-43 (1992)

269.   Tomljenovic, L.; Aluminum and Alzheimer's Disease: After a century of controversy, is there a plausible link?; J. Alzheimer's Disease, 23, 567-98 (2011)

270.   Arnold, S.E., et al.; The topographical and neuroanatomical distribution of neurofibrillary tangles and neuritic plaques in the cerebral cortex of patients with Alzheimer's disease; Cereb. Cortex; 1, 103-116 (1991)

271.   Hyman, B.T., et al.; Alzheimer's disease: Cell-specific pathology isolates the hippocampal formation; Science; 225:1168-70 (1984)

272.   Van Hoesen, G.W., et al.; Entorhinal cortex pathology in Alzheimer's disease; Hippocampus; 1:1-8 (1996)

273.   Gomez-Isla, T.; et al.; Profound loss of layer II entorhinal cortex neurons in very mild Alzheimer's disease; J. Neurosci.; 16:4491-4500 (1996)

274.   Coffey, C.E., et al.; Quantitative cerebral anatomy of the aging human brain; Neurology; Mar.; 42(3):527 (1992)

275.   Fjell, A.M., et al.; One-year brain atrophy evident in healthy aging; J. Neurosci.; Dec.; 29(48):15223-31 (2009)

276.   Van Landeghem, G.F., et al.; Aluminum speciation in cerebrospinal fluid of acutely aluminum-intoxicated dialysis patients before and after desferrioxamine treatment; a step in the understanding of the element's neurotoxicity; Nephrol. Dial. Transplant; 12:1692-98 (1997)

277.   Roberts, N.B., and Williams, P.; Silicon measurements in serum and urine by direct current plasma emission spectrometry; Clin. Chem.; 36(8):1480-85 (1990)

278.   Parry, R., et al.; Silicon and aluminum interactions in heamodialysis patients; Nephrol. Dial. Transplant; July; 13(7):1759-62 (1998)

279.   Reusche, E., and Seydel; Dialysis-associated encephalopathy: light and electron microscopic morphology and topography with evidence of aluminum by laser microprobe mass analysis; Acta Neuropathol.; 86:249-58 (1993)

280.   https://en.wikipedia.org/wiki/Apolipoprotein_E

281.   Van Exel, E., et al.; Effect of APOE ε4 allele on survival and fertility in an adverse environment; PLoS ONE; 12(7):e0179497 (2017)

282.   Drago, D., et al.; Potential pathogenic role of β-amyloid1-42-aluminum complex in Alzheimer's disease; Int. J. Biochem. Cell Biol.; 40:731-46 (2008)

283.   Gureje, O., et al.; APOE ε4 is not associated with Alzheimer's disease in elderly Nigerians; Ann. Neurol.; Jan.; 59(1):182-185 (2006)

284.   Hendrie, H.C., et al.; Incidence of dementia and Alzheimer's disease in 2 communities: Yoruba residing in Ibadan, Nigeria, and African Americans residing in Indianapolis, Indiana; JAMA; Feb.; 285(6):739-47 (2001)

285.   Awopetu, M.S., et al.; Water quality in a pipe distribution network: a case study of a communal water distribution network in Ibadan, Nigeria; WTI Transactions on Ecology and the Environment; 171:175-86 (2013)

286.   Adepoju, A.D., et al.; Preparation of silica from cassava periderm; J. Solid Waste Tech. Manag.; 42:216-21 (2016) Cassava peel was hand-sorted for pieces with brown periderm (approximately 5% of the cassava), was ashed at 600°C, and contained 61.5% silicate.

287.   Adebisi, J.A., et al.; Extraction of silica from cassava periderm using modified sol-gel method; Nigerian J. Tech. Dev.; June;15(2):57-65 (2018) TGA of periderm at 600°C results in 30% ash.

288.   Evans, E., et al.; Nigerian indigenous fermented foods: processes and prospects; Mycotoxin and food safety in developing countries; Chapter 7:153-80 (2013)

289.   Luo, Y., et al.; Altered expression of Abeta metabolism-associated molecules from D-galactose/AlCl(3) induced mouse brain; Mech. Ageing Dev. Apr.; 130(4):248-52 (2008)

290.   Sun, Z.Z., et al.; Alteration of Aβ metabolism-related molecules in predementia induced by AlCl3 and D-galactose; Age; 31:277-284 (2009)

291.   Drago, D.; Aluminum modulates effects of beta-amyloid1-42 on neuronal calcium homeostasis and mitochondrial functioning and is altered in a triple transgenic mouse model of Alzheimer's disease; Rejuvenation Reas.; 11(5):861-871 (2008)

292.   Erickson, K. I., Exercise training increases size of hippocampus and improves memory; PNAS; 108(7):3017-22 (2011)

293.   Xie, L., et al.; Sleep drives metabolite clearance from the adult brain; Science; Oct.; 342(6156) (2013)

294.   Leslie, J.G., et al.; Silicon in biological material. II. Variations in silicon contents in tissues of rat at different ages; Proc. Soc. Exp. Biol. Med.; 110:218- 20 (1962)

295.   Carlisle, E.M.; Silicon. In Biochemistry of the Essential Ultratrace Elements, Pp. 257-91, E. Frieden, ed. New York: Plenum Press (1984)

296.   Loeper, J., et al.; The physiological role of the silicon and its antiatheromatous action. In Biochemistry of Silicon and Related Problems, Pp. 281-96, G. Bendz and I Lindquist, eds. New York: Plenum Press (1978)

297.   https://www.cdc.gov/nchs/fastats/leading-causes-of-death.htm

298.   Schwarz, K., et al.; Inverse relation of silicon in drinking water and Atherosclerosis in Finland; Mar.; 309(8010):538-39 (1977)

299.   Gaballa, I.F., et al.; Dyslipidemia and disruption of L-carnitine in aluminum exposed workers; Egyptian J. Occup. Med.; 37(1):33-46 (2013) – There is a mistake in Table 2 of Gaballa's paper as in the text 5 people exposed to aluminum had a stroke while only 2 had monoplegia in the non-exposed group. Monoplegia has a number of causal factors, including stroke.

300.   Lemire, J., et al.; The disruption of L-carnitine metabolism by aluminum toxicity and oxidative stress promotes dyslipidemia in human astrocytic and hepatic cells; Toxicol. Lett. Jun.; 203(3):219-26 (2011)

301.   Pooyandjoo, M., et al.; The effect of (L-)carnitine on weight loss in adults: a systematic review and meta-analysis of randomized controlled trials; Obes. Rev.; Oct.; 17(10):970-6 (2016)

302.   Tipi-Akbas, P., et al.; Lowered serum total L-carnitine levels are associated with obesity at term pregnancy; J. Matern. Fetal Neonatal Med.; Oct.; 26(15):1479-83 (2013)

303.   Kurth, T., et al.; Body mass index and the risk of stroke in men; Arch. Intern. Med.; Dec.; 162:2557-62 (2002)

304.   Wald D.S., Law M., Morris J.K., Homocysteine and cardiovascular disease: evidence on causality from a meta-analysis. BMJ; 325(7374):1202 (2002)

305.   Ji Y., et al.; Vitamin B supplementation, homocysteine levels and the risk of cerebrovascular disease: a meta-analysis; Neurology (2013)

306.   Perry I.J., Refsum H., Morris R.W., Ebrahim S.B., Ueland P.M., Shaper A.G., Prospective study of serum total homocysteine concentration and risk of stroke in middle-aged British men. Lancet; 346:1395-8 (1995) Note: This decade long study of 5661 men 40-69 year of age shows that 107 men who had a stroke also had an average 2.8µM/L higher level of homocysteine as compared with men who did not have a stroke. These results compliment a study that showed a 10% decreased risk of recurrent stroke over a 2 year period with an average 3µM/L decrease in homocysteine levels resulting from vitamin supplementation[264].

307.   Toole J.F., Malinow M.R., Chambless L.E., Spence J.D., Pettigrew L.C., Howard V.J., Sides E.G., Wang C.H., Stampfer M.; Lowering homocysteine in patients with ischemic stroke to prevent recurrent stroke, myocardial infarction, and death; JAMA; 291: 565–575 (2004) Note: Based upon the data in this paper a 3µM/L drop in homocysteine due to B12 (6µg), B6 (200µg), and folic acid (20µg) daily supplementation resulted in 10% lower risk of recurrent stroke and a 16% lower risk of death on average among 1853 patients with non-disabling cerebral infarction but higher level (e.g. 100 fold) supplementation was ineffective.

308.   Censori B., Partziguian T., Manara O., Poloni M.; Plasma homocysteine and severe white matter disease; Neurol Sci; Oct.; 28(5):259-63 (2007)

309.   Sachdev P., Parslow R., Salonikas C., et al.; Homocysteine and the brain in midadult life: evidence for an increased risk of leukoaraiosis in men; Arch Neurol; Sep. 61(9): 1369-76 (2004)

310.   Chrysohoou, C., et al.; Aortic artery distensibility shows inverse correlation with heart rate variability in elderly non-hypertensive, cardiovascular disease-free individuals: the Ikaria Study; Heart Vessels; Jul.; 28(4):467-72 (2013)

311.   Gilbert-Barness, E., et al.; Aluminum toxicity; Arch Pediatr. Adolesc. Med.; 152:511-512 (1998)

312.   Walton, J.R.; Chronic aluminum intake causes Alzheimer's disease: Applying Sir Austin Bradford Hill's causality criteria; J. Alzheimer's Disease; 40:765-838 (2014) -See page 789

313.   Sorenson, J.R.J., et al.; Aluminum in the environment and human health; Environ. Health Perspectives; 8:3-95 (1974) - See top of page 44 and page 49 in this paper

314.   Besag, F.M.C.; Epilepsy in patients with autism: links, risks, and treatment challenges; Neuropsychiatric Dis. Treatment; 14:1-10 (2018)

315.   Mohammed, F.E.B., et al.; Assessment of hair aluminum, lead, and mercury in a sample of autistic Egyptian children: Environmental risk factors of heavy metals in autism; Behavioral Neurology; Article ID 545674:1-9 (2015)

316.   Bauman, M.L., and Kemper, T.L.; The neurobiology of autism; John Hopkins University Press; Structural Brain Anatomy in Autism: What is the Evidence? Chapt. 9:121-35 (2005)

317.   Papez, J.W.; A proposed mechanism for emotion; Arch Neuro. Psychiatry; 38:725-43 (1937)

318.   Howsman, D.P., et al.; Multivariate techniques enable a biochemical classification of children with autism spectrum disorder versus typically-developing peers: A comparison and validation study; Bioeng. Translational Med.; May; 1-10 (2018)

319.   Mailloux, R.J., Lemire, J., and Appanna, V.D.; Hepatic response to aluminum toxicity: dyslipidemia and liver diseases; Exp. Cell Res.; Oct.; 317(16):2231-8 (2011)

320.   Amiet, C., et al.; Epilepsy in autism is associated with intellectual disability and gender: evidence from a meta-analysis; Biol. Psychiatry; Osct.; 64(7):577-82 (2008)

321.   Kieth, L.S., et al.; Aluminum toxicokinetics regarding infant diet and vaccinations; Vaccine; May; 20 Suppl. 3:S13-7 (2002)

322.   Mitkus, R.J., et al.; Updated aluminum pharmacokinetics following infant exposures through diet and vaccination; Vaccine; Nov.; 29(51):0938-43 (2011)

323.   Tomljenovic, L., and Shaw, C.A.; Do aluminum vaccine adjuvants contribute to the rising prevalence of autism?; J. Inorg. Biochem.; 105:1489-99 (2011)

324.   Delong, G.; A positive association found between autism prevalence and childhood vaccination uptake across the U.S. population; J. Toxicol. Environ. Health A; 74(14):903-16 (2011)

325.   Lichtenstein, P., et al.; Environmental and heritable factors in the causation of cancer – Analyses of cohorts of twins from Sweden, Denmark, and Finland; N. Engl. J. Med.; 343-78-85 (2000)

326.   Bhandari, A., et al.; Colorectal cancer is a leading cause of cancer incidence and mortality among adults younger than 50 years in the UDA: a SEER-based analysis with comparison to other young-onset cancers; J. Investig. Med.; Feb.; 65(2):311-15 (2017)

327.   Siegel, R.L., et al.; Colorectal cancer incidence patterns in the United States, 1974-2013; J Natl. Cancer Inst.; 109(8):1-6 (2017) Breast cancer rate per 100,000 for U.S. women age 25-39: 1970 1.2, 1980 1.6, 1990 2.0, 2000 2.5, 2010 2.9

328.   Bingham, S.A., et al.; Dietary fibre in food and protection against colorectal cancer in the European Prospective Investigation into cancer and nutrition (EPIC): an observational study; The Lancet; May; 361:1496-1501 (2003)

329.   Fredholm, H., et al.; Breast cancer in young women: poor survival despite intensive treatment; PLoS One; Nov.; 4(11):e7695 (2009)

330.   Anders, C.K., et al.; Breast cancer before age 40 years; Semin Oncol.; June; 36(3):237-49 (2009)

331.   Johnson, R.H., et al.; Incidence of breast cancer with distant involvement among women in the United States, 1976-2009; JAMA, Feb., 309(8):800-5 (2013)

332.   Struewing, J.P., et al.; The risk of cancer associated with specific mutations of BRCA1 and BRCA2 among Ashkenazi Jews; N. Engl. J. Med.; 336:1401-8 (1997)

333.   https://en.wikipedia.org/wiki/Prostate_cancer

334.   World Cancer Report 2014; World Helath Organization; Chapter 5.11; ISBN 9283204298 (2014)

335.   Center, M.M., et al.; International variation in prostate cancer incidence and mortality rates; Eur. Urol.; June; 61(6):1079-92 (2012)

336.   Dickinson, J., et al.; Trends in prostate cancer incidence and mortality in Canada during the era of prostate-specific antigen screening; CMAJ Open; 4(1):E73-97 (2016) Prostate cancer incidence rate per 1,000 in 65-69 year old Canadian men: 1970 2.0, 1980 2.8, 1990 4.5, 2000 6.8, 2010 7.8

337.   Carlsen, E., et al.; Evidence for decreasing quality of semen during the past 50 years; BMJ; Sept.; 305:609-13 (1992)

338. Jorgensen, N., et al.; Coordinated European investigations of semen quality: results from studies of Scandinavian young men is a matter of concern; Int. J. Andrology; 29:54-61 (2006)

339. Levine, H., et al.; Temporal trends in sperm count: a systematic review and meta-regression analysis; Human Reproductive Update; Nov.; 23(6):646-59 (2017)

340. Bonde, J.P,, et al.; Relation between semen quality and fertility: a population-based study of 430 first-pregnancy planners; Lancet; Oct.; 352(9135):1172-7 (1998)

341. Martinez, C.S., et al.; Aluminum exposure for 60 days at human dietary levels impairs spermatogenesis and sperm quality in rats; Reproductive Toxicology; Oct.; 73:128-41 (2017)

342. Hickman, N., et al.; Effect of chronic administration of aluminum trichloride on testis among adult albino Wistar rats; J. Cytology and Histology; 4(5):1-4 (2013)

343. Miska-Schramm, A., et al.; The effect of aluminum exposure on reproductive ability in the bank vole (*Myodes glareolus*); Biol. Trace Elem. Res.; 177:97-106 (2017)

344. Klein, J.P., et al.; Aluminum content of human semen: Implications for semen quality; Reproductive Toxicology; 50:43-8 (2014)

345. Jamalan, M., et al.; Human sperm quality and metal toxicants: Protective effects of some flavonoids on male reproductive function; Int. J. Fertility Sterility; July-Sept.; 10(2):215-222 (2016)

346. Rahn, K., et al.; Cognitive impairment in multiple scelerosis: A forgotten disability remembered; Article online at: http://www.dana.org/news/cerebrum/detail.aspx?id=39986 Cerebrum; 1-19 (2012)

347. Compston, A. and Coles, A.; Multiple sclerosis; The Lancet; 372(9648):1502-17 (2008)

348. Clanet, M.; Jean-Martin Charcot. 1825 to 1893; International MS Journal; June; 15(2):59-61 (2008)

349. https://en.wikipedia.org/wiki/Multiple_sclerosis

350. Eldridge, W.A., et al.; Multiple sclerosis in twins; Neurology; Nov.; 30(11):1139-47 (1980)

351. Kurtzke, J.F.; Epidemiologic contributions to multiple sclerosis; Neurology; July; 30(7 Part 2):61-79 (1980)

352. Alonso, A., and Hernan, M.A.; Temporal trends in the incidence of multiple sclerosis – A systematic review; Neurology; July; 71(2):129-35 (2008)

353.	Cannell, J.J.; Autism and vitamin D; Med. Hypotheses; 70(4):750-9 (2008)

354.	Cannell, J.J.; Autism causes prevention and treatment; Sunrise River Press (2015)

355.	Azik, F.M., et al.; A different interaction between parathyroid hormone, calcitriol, and serum aluminum in chronic kidney disease; a pilot study; Int. Urol. Nephrol.; 43:467-70 (2011)

356.	https://www.hopkinsmedicine.org/healthlibrary/conditions/physical_medicine_and_rehab ilitation/multiple_sclerosis_and_pregnancy_85,P01160

357.	https://www.webmd.com/multiple-sclerosis/healthy-pregnancy-with-ms#1

358.	Benito-Leon, J.; Are the prevalence and incidence of multiple sclerosis changing?; Neuroepidemiology; 36:148-9 (2011)

359.	Hirst, C., et al.; Increasing prevalence and incidence of multiple sclerosis in South East Wales; J. Neurol. Neurosurg. Psychiatry; 80(4):386-91 (2008)

360.	Ribbons, K., et al.; Ongoing increase in incidence and prevalence of multiple sclerosis in Newcastle, Australia: A 50-year study; Multiple Sclerosis J.; 23(8):1063-71 (2017)

361.	Elhami, S.R., et al.; A 20-year incidence trend (1989-2008) and point prevalence (March 20, 2009) of multiple sclerosis in Tehran, Iran: a population-based study; Neuroepidemiology; 36(3):141-7 (2011)

362.	Golub, M.S., Han, B., Keen, C.L.; Aluminum uptake and effects on transferrin mediated iron uptake in primary cultures of rat neurons, astrocytes and oligodendrocytes; Neurotoxicology; Dec.; 20(6):961-70 (1999)

363.	Verstraeten, S.V., et al.; Myelin is a preferential target of aluminum-mediated oxidative damage; Arch. Biochem. Biophys.; 344:289-94 (1997)

364.	Itoh, M. et al.; Progressive leukoencephalopathy associated with aluminum deposits in myelin sheath; J. Child Neurology; 23(8):938-43 (2008)

365.	El-Aleem, S.A., et al.; Upregulation of the inducible nitric oxide synthase in rat hippocampus in a model of Alzheimer's disease: A possible mechanism of aluminum induced Alzheimer's; Egypt. J. Histol.; 32(1):173-180 (2008)

366.	Lukiw, W.J.; Nanomolar aluminum induces pro-inflammatory and pro-apoptotic gene expression in human brain cells in primary culture; J. Inorg. Biochem.; Sept.; 99(9):1895-8 (2005)

367.   Exley, C., et al.; Elevated urinary excretion of aluminium and iron in multiple sclerosis; Multiple Sclerosis; 12:533-40 (2006)

368.   Jones, K., et al.; Urinary excretion of aluminium and silicon in secondary progressive multiple sclerosis; EBioMedicine; 26:60-7 (2017)

369.   Mold, M., et al.; Aluminium in brain tissue in multiple sclerosis; Int. J. Environ. Res. Public Health; 15(8):1777 (2018) Including supplementary material p1-6 (2018)

370.   Scheller, N.M., et al.; Quadrivalent HPV vaccination and risk of multiple sclerosis and other demyelinating diseases of the central nervous system; JAMA; 313(1):54-61 (2015)

371.   Hu, Y.T, and Lopez-Alberola, R.; Two cases of pediatric multiple sclerosis after human papillomavirus vaccination; ACTRIMS Forum; San Diego, CA; Feb. 1-3; Abstract #P088 (2018)

372.   Dunstan, C.R., et al.; Effect of aluminum and parathyroid hormone on osteoblasts and bone mineralization in chronic renal failure; Calcified Tissue Int.; 36(1):133-38 (1984)

373.   Zafar, T.A., and Weaver, C.M.; Effects of aluminum on calcium absorption, growth, and bone calcium content; Int. J. Agri. Biol.; 1(3):138-41 (1999)

374.   Goodman, W., and O'Connor, J.; Aluminum alters calcium influx and efflux from bone in vitro; Kidney Int.; 39:602-7 (1991)

375.   Sprague, S.M., et al.; Aluminum inhibits bone nodule formation and calcification in vitro; Am. J. Physiol.; May; 264(Pt 2):F882-90 (1993)

376.   Murray, C.J.L., et al.; Global, regional, and national age-sex specific all-cause and cause-specific mortality for 240 causes of death, 1990-2013: a systematic analysis for the Global Burden of Disease Study 2013; Jan.; Lancet; 385(9963:177-71 (2015)

377.   Savica, R., et al.; Time trends in the incidence of Parkinson's disease; JAMA Neurology; 73(8):981-89 (2016)

378.   Gardner, R.C., et al.; Mild TBI and the risk of Parkinson's disease; May; 90(20):e1771-79 (2018)

379.   Hirsch, E.C., et al.; Iron and aluminum increase in the substantia nigra of patients with Parkinson's disease: an X-ray microanalysis; J. Neurochem.; Feb.; 56(2):446-51 (1991)

380.   Good, P.F., et al.; Neuromelanin-containing neurons of the substantia nigra accumulate iron and aluminum in Parkinson's disease: a LAMMA study; Oct.; 593(2):343-6 (1992)

381. Fitzgerald, K., Lead (aluminum) and homocysteine levels in a series of individuals diagnosed with Parkinson's disease: https://www.drkarafitsgerald.com/2014/04/16/ (2014)

382. VanDuyn, N., et al.; The metal transporter SNF-3/DMT-1 mediates aluminum-induced dopamine neuron degeneration; J. Neurochem.; Jan.; 124(1):147-57 (2013)

383. Ke, Y., et al.; Age-dependent and iron-independent expression of two mRNA isoforms of divalent metal transporter 1 in rat brain; Neurobiol. Aging; 26:739-48 (2005)

384. Salazar, J., et al.; Divalent metal transporter 1 (DMT1) contributes to neurodegeneration in animal models of Parkinson's disease; PNAS; Nov.; 105(47):18578-18583 (2008)

385. Junwei, D.I. and Shuping, B.I.; Aluminum facilitation of the iron-mediated oxidation of DOPA to melanin; Anal. Sci.; Apr.; 20:629-34 (2004)

386. Wilczek, A. and Mishima, Y.; Inhibitory effects of melanin monomers, dihydroxyindole-2-carboxylic acid (DHICA) and dihydroxyindole (DHI) on mammalian tyrosinase, with special reference to the role of DHICA/DHI ratio in melanogenesis; Pigment Cell Res.; Apr.; 8(2):105-12 (1995)

387. Sanchez-Iglesias, S., et al.; Brain oxidative stress and selective behavior of aluminum in specific areas of rat brain: potential effects in a 6-OHDA-induced model of Parkinson's disease; J. Neurochem.; May; 109(3):879-88 (2009)

388. Jenner, P., et al.; Oxidative stress as a cause of nigral cell death in Parkinson's disease and incidental Lewy body disease; Ann. Neurol.; 32:S82-7 (1992)

389. Zucca, F.A., et al.; Neuromelanin of the human substratia nigra: an update; Neurotox. Res.; Jan.; 25(1):13-23 (2014)

390. Zecca, L., et al.; Iron, neuromelanin, and ferritin content in the substantia nigra of normal subjects at different ages: consequences for iron storage and neurodegenerative processes; J. Neurochem, 76:1766-73 (2001)

391. Zecca, L., et al.; Substrata nigra neuromelanin: structure, synthesis, and molecular behavior; J. Clin. Pathol: Mol. Pathol.; 54:414-418 (2001) Unpublished results see page 416.

392. Bouasla, I., et al.; Antioxidant effect of alpha lipoic acid on hepatotoxicity induced by aluminum chloride in rats; Int. J. Pharm. Sci. Rev. Res.; Dec.; 29(2):19-25 (2014)

393. Joshua, J., et al.; Anti-inflammatory drugs and risk of Parkinson disease; Neurology; Mar.; 74(12):995-1002 (2010)

394.   Patterson, D. Molecular genetic analysis of Down syndrome; Human Genetics; July; 126(1):195-214 (2009)

395.   Moore, P.B., et al.; Gastrointestinal absorption of aluminum is increased in Downs syndrome; Biol. Psychiatry; Feb.; 15:41(4):488-92 (1997)

396.   Lai, F. and Williams, R.S.; A prospective study of Alzheimer's disease in Down syndrome; Arch Neurol.; 46:849-53 (1989)

397.   Wilcock, D.M., and Griffin, W.S.; Down's syndrome, neuroinflammation and Alzheimer's neuropathogenesis; J. Neuroinflammation; 10:84 (2013)

398.   House, E., et al.; Aluminum, iron, and copper in human brain tissues donated to the Medical Research Council's cognitive functioning and ageing study; Metallomics; Jan. 4(1):56-65 (2012)

399.   Moore, P.B.; et al.; Absorption of aluminum-26 in Alzheimer's disease, measured using accelerator mass spectrometry; 11:66-69 (2000)

400.   Taylor, G.A., et al.; Gastrointestinal absorption of aluminum in Alzheimer's disease: response to aluminum citrate; Age Ageing; Mar.; 21(2):81-90 (1992)

401.   Hartley, D., et al.; Down syndrome and Alzheimer's disease: Common pathways and common goals; Alzheime's Dement.; June; 11(6):700-709 (2015)

402.   Sillanpaa, M., et al.; Temporal changes in the incidence of epilepsy in Finland: Nationwide study; Epilepsy Res.; 71:206-15 (2006)

403.   Fiest, K.M., et al.; Prevalence and incidence of epilepsy - A systematic review and meta-analysis of international studies; Neurology; 88:296-303 (2017)

404.   Camfield, C.S., et al.; Death in children with epilepsy: a population-based study; Lancet; June; 359(9321):1891-5 (2002)

405.   Callenbach, P.M., et al.; Mortality risk in children with epilepsy: the Dutch study of epilepsy in childhood; Pediatrics; June; 107(6):1259-63 (2001)

406.   Kopeloff, L.M., et al.; Chronic experimental epilepsy in Macaca mulatta; Neuology, 4:218-227 (1954)

407.   Soper, V., et al.; Chronic alumina temporal lobe seizures in monkeys; Exp. Neurology; Oct.; 62(1):99-121 (1978)

408.   David, J., et al.; Behavioral and electrical correlates of absence seizures induced by thalamic stimulation in juvenile rhesus monkeys with frontal aluminum hydroxide implants: A pharmacologic evaluation; J. Pharmacological Methods; May; 7(3):219-229 (1982)

409.   Ward, A.A.; Topical convulsant metals. In: Experimental models of epilepsy. A manual for the laboratory worker, eds. D.P. Purpura, et al.; pp.13-35 New York: Raven Press (1972)

410.   Alfey, A.C.; Aluminum toxicity in patients with chronic renal failure; Ther. Drug Monit.; 15:593-97 (1993)

411.   Elger, C.E., et al.; Therapeutic problems in patients suffering from aluminum encephalopathy; Neuroimmunologie spinale krankenheiten neuropsychologie metalische enzephalopathien neurologische notfalle interventionelle neuroradiologie verhandlungen der deutschen gesellschaft fur neurologie; 4; K. Poeck, et al. editors; Springer (1987)

412.   Glenn, C.M., et al.; Dialysis-associated seizures in children and adolescents; Pediatr. Nephrol.; 6(2):182 (1992)

413.   Freiman, S.B., et al.; Seizure and elevated blood aluminum in a remelt furnace operator: connection of coincidence?; Am. J. Emergency Med.; May; 23(3):419-20 (2005)

414.   Hantson, P.H., et al.; Encephalopathy with seizures after use of aluminum-containing bone cement; Lancet; Dec.; 344:1647 (1994)

415.   CDC Centers for Disease Control and Prevention; Vaccines and Preventable Diseases; https://www.cdc.gov/vaccines/vpd/should-not-vacc.html

416.   Mittal, M., et al.; Reactive oxygen species in inflammation and tissue repair; Antioxidants Redox Signalling; 20(7):1126-67 (2014)

417.   Exley, C.; The Pro-oxidant activity of aluminum; Free Radical Biol. Med.; 36(3):380-87 (2004)

418.   Kong, S., et al.; Aluminum III facilitates the oxidation of NADH by the superoxide anion; Free Radical Biol. Med.; 13(1):79-81 (1992)

419.   Pogue, A.I., et al.; Characterization of an NF-kappaB-regulated, miRNA-146a-mediated down-regulation of complement factor H(CFH) in metal-sulfate stressed human brain cells; J. Inorg. Biochem.; Nov.; 103(11):1591-5 (2009)

420.   Lawrence, T.; The nuclear factor NF-κB pathway in inflammation; Cold Spring Harb. Perspect. Biol.; 1:a001651 (2009)

421. Tsunoda, M., and Sharma, R.P.; Modulation of tumor necrosis factor alpha expression in mouse brain after exposure to aluminum in drinking water; Arch. Toxicol.; Nov.; 73(8-9):419-26 (1999)

422. Wilcox, B.J., et al.; FOXO3A genotype is strongly associated with human longevity; PNAS; Sept.; 105(37):13987-92 (2008)

423. Grossi, V., et al.; The longevity SNP rs2802292 uncovered: HSF1 activates stress-dependent expression of FOXO3 through an intronic enhancer; Nucl. Acids Res.; 46(11):5587-5600 (2018)

424. Xu, D., et al.; Homocysteine accelerates endothelial cell senescence; FEBS Letters; 470:20-24 (2000)

425. Santos, J.H., et al.; Mitochondrial hTERT exacerbates free-radical-mediated mtDNA damage; Aging Cell; 3:399-411 (2004)

426. Seaborn, C.D., and Nielsen, F.H.; Silicon deprivation decreases collagen formation in wounds and bone, and ornithine transaminase enzyme activity in liver; Biol. Trace Elem. Res.; 89(3):251-61 (2002).

427. Seaborn, C.D., et al.; Silicon: A nutritional beneficence for bones, brains and blood vessels?; Nutrition Today; Jul./Aug.; 1993:13-8 (1993)

428. Schwarz, K.; A bound form of silicon in glycosaminoglycans and polyuronides; Proc. Natl. Acad. Sci. U.S.A.; 70(5):1608-12 (1973)

429. Aranjo, L.A., et al.; Use of silicon for skin and hair care: an approach of chemical forms available and efficacy; An. Bras. Dermatol.; 91(3):331-5 (2016)

430. Richman, E.L., et al.; Choline intake and risk of lethal prostate cancer: incidence and survival; Am. J. Clin. Nutr.; 96:855-63 (2012)

431. Aguilar, F., et al.; Calcium silicate and silicon dioxide/silica acid gel added for nutritional purposes to food supplements; EFSA J.; 1132:1-24 (2009)

432. Aguilar, F., et al.; Choline-stabilized orthosilicic acid added for nutritional purposes to food supplements; EFSA J.; 948:1-23 (2009)

433. Jacqmin-Gadda, H., et al.; Components of drinking water and risk of cognitive impairment in the elderly; Am. J. Epidemiol.; 139:48-57 (1994)

434. Iler, R.K.; Soluble silicates; ACS Symposium Series, 194(7):95-114 (1982)

435.   Alexander, G.B.; The reaction of low molecular weight silicic acids with molybdic acid; J. Am. Chem. Soc.; 75:5655-57 (1975)

436.   Taylor, P.D., et al.; Soluble silica with high affinity for aluminum under physiological and natural conditions; J. Am. Chem. Soc.; 119, 8852-56 (1997)

437.   Jugdaohsingh, R., et al.; High-aluminum-affinity silica is a nanoparticle that seeds secondary aluminosilicate formation; PLOS; Dec. 13, (2013)

438.   Kozisek, F.; Health risks from drinking demineralized water; National Institute of Public Health, Czech Republic; Chapter 12; Water, sanitation, and health protection and the human environment; W.H.O.; Geneva (2005)

439.   Dietzel, M.; Dissolution of silicates and the stability of polysilicic acid; Geochimica et Cosmochimica Acta; 64(19):3275-81 (2000)

440.   Schlottmann, U.; Soluble Silicates; OECD SIDS Initial Assessment Report for SIAM 18; UNEP Publications; Paris, France; April 20-23 (2004)

441.   Flythe, J.E., et al.; Silicate nephrolithiasis after ingestion of supplements containing silica dioxide; Am. J. Kidney Dis.; July; 54(1):127-30 (2009)

442.   Lai, J.C., et al.; Inhibition of glycolysis by aluminum; J. Neurochem.; 42:438-46 (1984)

443.   Casey, R., et al.; Silicon in beer and brewing; J. Sci. Food Agric.; 90:784-788 (2010)

444.   Pogue, A.I., et al.; Selective targeting and accumulation of aluminum in tissue of C57BL/6J mice fed aluminum sulfate activates a pro-inflammatory NK-kB-microRNA-146a signaling program; J. Neurology Neuro Toxicol.; 1(1)1-10 (2017)

445.   Exley, C., et al.; Aluminum in tobacco smoke and cannabis and smoking related disease; Am. J. Med.; 118:276 (2006)

446.   Flarend, R.E., et al.; A preliminary study of the dermal absorption of aluminum from antiperspirants using aluminum-26: Food Chem. Toxicol.; Feb.; 39(2):163-8 (2001)

447.   Stevens, L., et al.; Amounts of artificial food dyes in foods and sweets commonly consumed by children; Clin. Pediatr.; Apr., published online (2014)

448.   Sirnivasan, P.T., et al.; Aluminum in drinking water: an overview; Water SA; Jan.; 25(1):47-56 (1999)

449.   Palazzolo, D.L., et al.; Trace metals derived from electronic cigarette (ECIG) generated aerosol: potential problem of ECIG devices that contain nickel; Frontiers in Physiol.; Jan.; 7:1-17 Article 663 (2017)

450.   Bassioni, G., et al.; Risk assessment of using aluminum foil in food preparation, Int. J. Electrochem. Sci.; 7:4498-4509 (2012)

451.   Flarend, R.E., et al.; In vivo absorption of aluminum-containing vaccine adjuvants using 26Al; Vaccine; Aug.-Sept.; 15(12-13):1314-8 (1997)

452.   The future of aluminium; Spectator; July; 71:76-77 (1893)

453.   Pearl, J. and Mackenzie, D.; The book of why – The new science of cause and effect; Basic Books; NY,NY (2018)

454.   Wahls, T. and Adamson, E.; The Wahls Protochol: A radical new way to treat all chronic autoimmune conditions using paleo principles; Avery; Penguin Group, NY, NY (2014)

455.   Geier, D.A., et al.; A prospective study of transsulfuration biomarkers in autistic disorders; Neurochem. Res.; Feb.; 34(2):386-93 (2009)

456.   De Los Santos, J., et al.; Elimination of sulfates from wastewaters by natural aluminosilicate modified with uric acid; Resource-Efficient Tech.; 1:98-105 (2015)

457.   Waring, R.H.; Report on absorption of magnesium sulfate (Epsom salts) across the skin; http://www.epsomsaltcouncil.org/wp-content/uploads/2015/10/report_on_absorption_of_magnesium_sulfate.pdf

458.   Mandriota, S.J., et al.; Aluminum chloride promotes tumorigenesis and metastasis in normal murine mammary gland epithelial cells; Int. J. Cancer; 139:2781-90 (2016)

459.   Linhard, C.; et al.; Use of underarm cosmetic products in relation to risk of breast cancer: A case-control study; EBioMedicine; 21:79-85 (2017)

460.   Adachi, H., et al.; Plasma homocysteine levels and atherosclerosis in Japan; Epidemiological study by use of carotid ultrasonography; Stroke; Sept.; 33:2177-81 (2002)

461.   Deng, Q., et al.; Understanding the association between environmental factors and longevity in Hechi, China: A drinking water and soil quality perspective; Int. J. Environ. Res. Public Health; 15:2272:1-17 (2018)

462.   Yang, J.; An analysis of the longevous population in Bama; Chin. J. Popul. Sci.; 4(4):351-6 (1992)

463.   Xiao, Z., et al.; Solving the mystery of the status and longevity of centenarians in Bama; Chin. J. Popul. Sci.; 8(4):385-94 (1996)

464.   Song, W., et al.; Public health in China: An environmental and socioeconomic perspective; March; 129:9-17 (2016)

465. Deng, Q., et al.; Understanding the natural and socioeconomic factors behind regional longevity in Guangxi, China: Is the centenarian ratio a good enough indicator for assessing the longevity phenomenon? Int. J. Environ. Res. Public Health; 15:938:1-16 (2018)

466. Zhang, N,, et al.; Study on regional distribution of longevity and the hair's chemical elements content of the crowds in Bama county, Guangxi province; Clin. J. Gerontol.; 9, 050 (2010)

467. Liang, Z.; Understanding the longevity phenomenon in Bama; China Stat.; (2004)

468. Hu, H., et al.; Depositional chemistry of chert during the late Paleozoic from western Guangxi and its implication for the tectonic evolution of the Youjiang Basin; Sci. China Earth Sci.; March; doi: 10.1007/s11430-012-4496-y (2012)

469. Qiu, Z., et al.; Geochemistry and sedimentary background of the Middle-Upper Permian cherts in the Xiang-Qian-Gui region; Acta. Petrol. Sin.; 26:3612-28 (2010)

470. Murray, R.W., et al.; Diagenetic formation of bedded chert: Evidence from chemistry of the chert-shale coupler; Geology; 20:271-4 (1992)

471. Bustillo, M.A.; Chapter 3 Silicification of continental carbonates; Dev. Sedimentology; Dec.; 62 doi: 10.1016/S0070-4571(09)06203-7 (2010)

472. Martin, W.R. and Sayles, F.L.; The recycling of biogenic material at the seafloor; Section 7.02.6.1 Dissolved silica profiles in pore waters; Treatise on Geochemistry; (2003).

473. Epoch Times; Bama: Land of Longevity; Aug. 30 (2013)

474. Heckman, J.R., et al.; Pumpkin yield and disease response to amending soil with silicon; Hort. Sci.; 38(4):552-4 (2003)

475. Rawat, K., et al.; Quantitative assessment of silicon in fresh and processed bamboo shoots and its potential as functional element in food, nutraceuticals, and cosmeceuticals; https://worldbamboo.net/wbcxi/papers/Rawat,%20Kanchan,%20Nirmala%20Chongtham,%20M.S.%20Bisht.pdf

476. Nordal, K.P., et al.; Aluminum overload a predisposing condition for epileptic seizures in renal-transplant patients treated with Cyclosporin; Lancet; 2:153-4 (1985)

477. Mold, M., et al.; Aluminum in brain tissue in epilepsy: A case report from Camelford; Int. J. Environ. Res. Pub. Health; 16(2129):1-11 (2019)

478. Di Lorenzo, F. and Di Lorenzo, B.; Iron and aluminum in Alzheimer's disease; Neuroendrocrinol. Lett.; 34:504-7 (2013)

479.   Auvin, S., et al.; Altered vaccine-induced immunity in children with Dravet syndrome; Epilepsia; 59:e45-e50 (2018)

480.   Schuiling, R.D., and Tickell, O.; Olivine against climate change and ocean acidification; http://www.innovationconcepts.eu/res/literatuurSchuiling/olivineagainstclimatechange23.pdf

481.   Popplewell, J.F., et al.; Kinetics of uptake and elimination of silicic acid by a human subject: a novel application of 32Si and accelerator spectrometry; J. Inorg. Biochem.; Feb.; 15:69(3):177-80 (1998)

482.   Kavak, D.D., et al.; Investigation of structural properties of clinoptilolite rich zeolites in simulated digestive conditions and their cytotoxicity against Caco-2 cells in vitro; J. Porous Materials; April, 1-8 (2012)

483.   FROXIMUN F&E; Safety and efficiency evidence of the MANC; Test report on the examination of the long-term application of natural zeolite; Preliminary Version; Table 2 and Table 3; Feb.; (2016)

484.   Sirotiak, M., et al.; Sorption kinetics of selected heavy metals adsorption to natural and Fe(III) modified zeolite tuff containing clinoptilolite mineral, Research Paper – Slovak University of Technology, Bratislava; 23(36):41-7 (2015)

485.   Edwards, D.; FDA U.S. Food & Drug Admin.; Re: GRAS Notice No. AGRN-25, Letter to Thomas Bergen, V.P.; G-Sciences; May 4 (2018)

486.   Mold, M., et al.; Aluminum and amyloid-B in familial Alzheimer's disease; J. Alz. Dis.; 1:1-8 (2019)

487.   McLachlan, D.R.C., et al.; Aluminum in neurological disease – a 36 year multicenter study; J. Alzheimer's Dis. Parkinsonism; 8:457 (2018)

488.   Linhart, C., et al.; Aluminum in brain tissue in non-neurodegenerative / non-neurodevelopmental disease: A comparison with multiple sclerosis; Exposure and Health; Feb.; https://doi.org/10.1007/s12403-020-00346-9 (2020)

489.   Jurkic, L.M.; et al.; Biological and therapeutic effects of ortho-silicic acid and some ortho-silicic acid-releasing compounds: New perspectives for therapy; Nutr. Metab.; 10(2):1-12 (2013)

490.   Silva, V.S., and Goncalves, P.P., The inhibitory effect of aluminium on the (Na+/K+)ATPase activity of rat brain cortex synaptosomes; J. Inorg. Biochem.; Sep.; 97(1):143-50 (2003)